HEALTHY EATING
DIABETES

Delicious recipes for type 2 diabetes

Authors: Doris Fritzsche, Marlisa Szwillus

Photography: Sudio L'Eveque

CONTENTS

TYPE 2 DIABETES … 4

Type 2 diabetes – diagnosis: diabetes … 6

Controlling diabetes –
the fundamentals of treatment
    Diet and exercise
    education and advice … 8

Type 2 diabetes – I still have some questions…
    Typical and atypical symptoms –
    recognising problems and reacting … 10

Losing weight – and living lighter
    More exercise everyday and
    reducing the energy intake … 12

Carbohydrates – the lowdown
for carbohydrate exchanges (CE) … 14

Glycemic index and glycemic load
    more indexes… … 16

Everyday eating – without the worry
    Eating a diabetic-friendly diet
    is actually quite easy … 18

Eating and drinking – staying nourished throughout the day
    From the start into the day via eating in restaurants and
    canteens to late meals … 20

RECIPES … 22

Breakfast, Snacks and Drinks

Muesli with fresh fruit … 24

Citrus fruit muesli, Fresh grain muesli … 26

Apple & coconut porridge, Hearty millet muesli … 27

Bread roll with basil tofu,
Corned beef open sandwich … 28

Cheese & apricot open sandwich,
Apple & cream cheese open sandwich … 29

Hummus with sesame seeds … 30

Eggplant spread with capsicum
Olive & roasted vegetable paste … 31

Zucchini scrambled eggs,
Cheese & vegetable snack … 32

Cheese & salad rolls,
Capsicum boats with tzatziki … 33

Ham rolls with radishes,
Herring salad on wholegrain bread … 34

Indian lassi, Vegetable drink … 36

Peach frappé with cream,
Vanilla & ginger tea … 37

Snacks and Starters

Bean salad with tuna … 38

Chicory & grape salad with cheese dressing,
Warm savoy cabbage salad … 40

Chickpea salad with herb dressing,
Couscous salad … 42

Moroccan carrot salad … 44

Vegetable salad with yoghurt,
Orange salad with onions … 45

Red lentil soup with parsley oil,
Barley & vegetable soup … 46

Jerusalem artichoke soup, French onion soup … 48

Asian vegetable soup, Quick tomato soup … 50

Warm radicchio salad, Broccoli with walnuts … 52

Mediterranean vegetables,
Cauliflower with a curried yoghurt sauce … 54

Fennel & tomatoes with Parmesan,
Spinach in a sesame sauce … 56

Eggplant bake, Kohlrabi & potato bake … 58

Cheesy zucchini parcels, Savoury baked apples … 60

Main Courses – Vegetarian

Vegetable rice with hard-boiled eggs	62
Spinach dumplings with tomato sauce, Millet with ratatouille	64
Cabbage rolls with bulgur filling	66
Spaghetti with pumpkin seed & herb pesto, Spinach-filled cannelloni	68
Pizza with artichokes	70
Wok vegetables with glass noodles, Fried vegetables with parsley sauce	72
Turnip quiche	74
Lentil rice with vegetables	76

Main Courses – With Fish

Mackerel baked in foil	78
Fish with panfried mushrooms, Cod with leek and tomatoes	80
Fish fillets in a sesame crust	82
Barramundi in an olive and caper sauce, Fish kebabs with lemon sauce	84
Ocean perch ragout	86
Capsicum barley with prawns, Ling fillet in a cheese & vegetable crust	88
Salmon on Waldorf salad	90
Barramundi & vegetables, Fish osso buco	92

Main Courses – With Poultry

Creole chicken casserole	94
Filled turkey rolls, Curried turkey strips	96
Chicken breast with pineapple, Duck breast with broccoli and nuts	98
Lemon chicken, Oven-baked turkey drumstick	100

Main Courses – With Meat

Lasagne with meat and vegetables	102
Burgers with roasted vegetables	104
Eggplant pasta with prosciutto, Venison medallions with a herb crust	106
Spicy lamb pilaf	108

Desserts and Baking

Pancakes with plum compote	110
Red berry jelly with a yoghurt sauce, Marinated peaches with cream cheese	112
Cherry & pumpernickel cup, Poached chocolate pears	114
Moroccan oranges, Strawberry & tofu ice cream	116
Raspberry jelly with coconut cream, Yoghurt & orange muffins	118
Cream cheese croissants with poppy seeds	120
Cinnamon apple crumble, Cheesecake with apricots	122

LOOK IT UP

The food pyramid	124
Weekly diet plan	126
Recipes index – by chapter	129
Index	130
Imprint	132

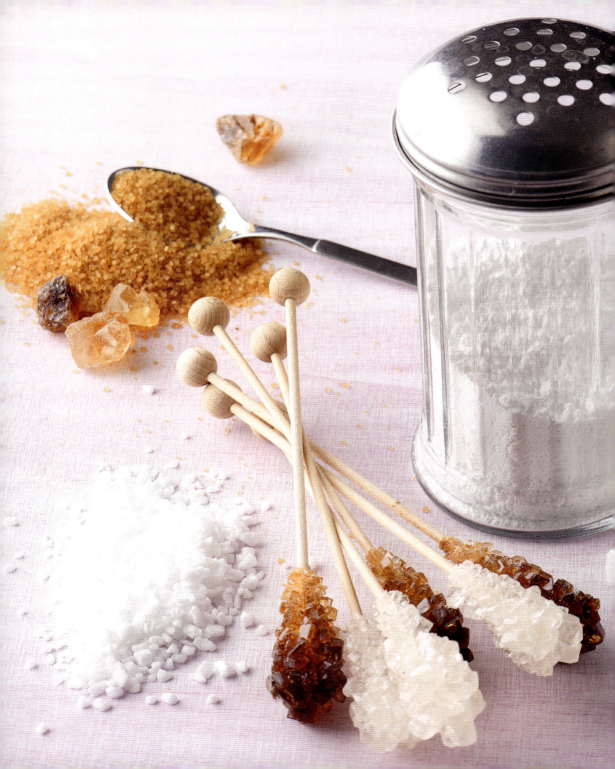

TYPE 2 DIABETES
WHEN INSULIN DOESN'T WORK

Approximately two million Australians have diabetes and most of them are diagnosed with type 2. This number is growing steadily, with cases now appearing increasingly in younger patients.

Have you just been diagnosed with diabetes? Don't panic; you're not the only one. More and more people of all ages have high blood glucose levels. Permanently changing your diet is the most effective basic treatment to prevent any further complications, making it easier to live with the metabolic disorder known as type 2 diabetes, a form of diabetes mellitus.

This book will provide you with answers to many important questions, helping you with your everyday life and dietary changes. It also contains a number of hints and tips for buying groceries, as well as delicious new recipes for your enjoyment.

TYPE 2 DIABETES
DIAGNOSIS: DIABETES

WHEN PEOPLE WITH DIABETES eat food containing starch and sugar, their blood glucose levels increase much more than those of people with a healthy sugar metabolism. If these levels exceed a set threshold, sugar is eliminated in the urine through the kidneys. This elimination of sugar is detectable when blood glucose levels are between 180 and 200 milligrams per 100 millilitres (10 to 11.1 millimoles per litre). The official name for the disease is diabetes mellitus; "diabetes" comes from a Greek word meaning "that which passes through" and "mellitus", which is derived from the Latin word for honey.

WHY ARE BLOOD GLUCOSE LEVELS HIGHER?

Blood glucose levels may be higher in diabetics if insulin is no longer produced or not produced in sufficient amounts by the body. Insulin is a pancreatic hormone and performs one of the most important roles in metabolising sugar: it "opens" the body's cells to allow the glucose to enter, thus providing nutrients and energy to the body. If this hormone is lacking or unable to function properly, two critical problems arise: the body's cells are not properly supplied with the energy they require, and the blood sugar content rises excessively, itself causing a condition known as a glucose intolerance. The increase in blood glucose levels happens gradually, and often remains undetected and undiagnosed for a long time.

TYPICAL SYMPTOMS

Type 2 diabetes frequently goes undetected for long periods of time, because the initial symptoms of consistently high blood glucose levels are usually very vague and are not immediately associated with diabetes. Typical symptoms include for example fatigue and lethargy, excessive thirst and frequent urination.

If proper blood glucose treatment is received, these symptoms will soon subside. If they are left untreated, however, elevated blood glucose levels can eventually lead to other complications, in particular those affecting the vascular and nervous system.

TYPE 1 OR TYPE 2?

If blood glucose rises to an extremely high level, this metabolic status can cause an intense loss of consciousness, known as a diabetic coma. This only poses a serious risk to diabetics who cannot produce any insulin in their pancreas at all, which is why treatment of type 1 diabetes involves the injection of insulin. With type 2 diabetes, the pancreas produces a sufficient amount of insulin, at least in the early stages of the illness. However, the cells' resistance to the insulin means the hormone cannot function properly, causing blood glucose levels to slowly rise.

WHAT IS THE TREATMENT FOR TYPE 2 DIABETES?

Most people with type 2 diabetes tend to be overweight, which strengthens the insulin resistance and further hinders the hormone's ability to function correctly. For this reason, treatment of type 2 diabetes is always initially based on action to reduce body weight (see pages 8 and 12).

Generally adjusting various eating habits and moderately increasing physical activity are thus the preferred methods for improving insulin function and regaining control of the elevated blood glucose levels.

A CHANGE IN LIFESTYLE

Being diagnosed with diabetes may encourage you to improve your wellbeing by adopting a more active lifestyle and being more aware of your diet generally. Healthy eating will boost your quality of life by ensuring an optimum supply of vitamins, minerals, dietary fibre and bioactive plant compounds.

You will soon find that this will also be reflected in clear skin, healthy nails, glossy hair and better moods overall. Having to change your eating habits because of diabetes does not mean depriving yourself or going on boring diets, but rather eating colourful, varied and delicious "good mood food".

Those who also ensure they get sufficient exercise will strengthen their muscles and immune system, train their cardiovascular system and promote healthy stress management. Physical activities similarly help with losing and maintaining weight (see the suggestions on page 8 relating to this topic). Sometimes it's just a question of making a more conscious effort to exercise in everyday life and to move more. Why not take the stairs instead of the lift, or get off at a bus stop slightly further away?

WHEN DOES TYPE 2 DIABETES HAVE TO BE TREATED WITH MEDICATION?

It is often advisable to treat type 2 diabetes with medication if a change in lifestyle proves to be insufficient to normalise the blood glucose levels in the body. Ask your doctor if this is the case for you and when you should start taking medications to assist with the changes in your diet and exercise regime.

MINI DIABETES DICTIONARY

BLOOD GLUCOSE/SUGAR: The volume of sugar (glucose) in the blood. The standard levels are between 60 and 140 milligrams per 100 millilitres (3.3 to 7.8 millimoles per litre).

DIABETES MELLITUS: A metabolic disorder characterised by high blood glucose.
Type 1 diabetes = insulin-dependent diabetes mellitus
Type 2 diabetes = non-insulin-dependent diabetes mellitus

GLUCOSE INTOLERANCE: Glucose, formed by sugar and starch, cannot infiltrate the cells as required. This causes an above-average rise in blood glucose levels.

INSULIN: A hormone produced in the pancreas which allows blood glucose to enter the cells. Various forms of insulin are now manufactured and available to treat diabetes.

INSULIN RESISTANCE: The body's "resistance" to insulin. In the case of type 2 diabetes, this resistance is intensified by excess weight and lack of exercise.

URINE GLUCOSE: Sugar/glucose eliminated in the urine because the blood glucose levels are so high that the kidneys can no longer retain the sugar.

CONTROLLING DIABETES

THE FUNDAMENTALS OF TREATMENT

THE MOST IMPORTANT THING when treating diabetes is to ensure maximum quality of life. This includes individual adjustment of blood glucose levels to prevent acute and chronic health complications resulting from diabetes. Successful treatment of the disease is based on several main aspects, which will allow you to achieve this goal.

THE 6 PILLARS OF TREATMENT

> diet
> exercise
> training and advice
> self-checks
> medical checks
> medication

DIET AND EXERCISE

Changing one's diet should permanently normalise body weight and take the strain off the pancreas. You can gradually achieve this goal by adopting a varied diet which distributes carbohydrate intake evenly throughout the day (see page 15) and gives preference to foods with low glycemic load (see page 16). You should also reduce your fat intake, pay attention to good fat quality, and give preference to high-quality vegetable oils (e.g. rapeseed oil, olive oil). This similarly enables you to positively influence blood lipids. In this way, you have the capacity to create the perfect basis for maintaining your wellbeing as well as a healthy metabolism.

Apart from dietary changes, regular and sustained physical activity is the most effective way to not only treat type 2 diabetes but to also give other positive health benefits.

TRAINING AND ADVICE

A book cannot replace an individual consultation with a doctor or dietitian. Many medical practices, diabetes specialists and diabetes centres hold special training courses and mentoring sessions for diabetics, where you will receive personalised instruction tailored to your treatment needs. Many issues can be discussed there, and you will also be given many helpful tips on how to live with diabetes generally, and how to avoid the pitfalls associated with a new diet or exercise regime.

MEDICAL CHECKS

Above all, you must go regularly for all the recommended medical check-ups, as this allows possible complications to be detected early on and treated quickly before they have a serious effect on your health. Diabetes Australia and the NDSS (National Diabetes Services Scheme) will advise you on how often and which check-ups are required to monitor your health.

MEDICATION

If blood glucose levels cannot be adequately reduced by diet and exercise alone, medication may be required (either temporarily or permanently). However this must not be considered as a substitute for eating a balanced diet and exercising regularly – it is important to continue to make these changes as well.

Many different active ingredients with varying impacts on metabolism are available in tablet form to treat type 2 diabetes. Insulin is increasingly being administered in the early stages of this disease, for example if the body's insulin reserves are sufficient to cope in between meals, but the body can no longer produce enough of its own insulin at meal times.

IDENTIFYING AND ELIMINATING HYPOGLYCEMIA

Hypoglycemia is the term used to describe the condition when blood glucose drops to less than 80 milligrams per 100 millilitres (4.4 millimoles per litre). To counteract this, the body releases hormones (glucagon, adrenalin and others) which can raise these levels. The symptoms of hypoglycemia vary from one person to another, and often depend on how quickly the blood glucose drops. The most important thing is to know what these symptoms are and to act immediately as soon as they become apparent, whether in yourself or in someone you know.

The typical symptoms of a rapid drop in blood glucose are a sudden and ravenous appetite, cold sweats, striking pallor, shivers, palpitations or feelings of anxiety.

For slower drops in blood glucose, the symptoms are often not as clear, and can include any of the following: slight headaches, visual impairments (double vision), difficulties with routine actions, and unexplained annoyance, and possibly aggression.

Make sure your family members, friends and colleagues are aware of the typical symptoms you may show, and ask them to help immediately if you start showing any of them. It is important to act straightaway to prevent severe hypoglycemia, that is, a loss of consciousness.

How to treat hypoglycemia: sit or lie down. Take 4 glucose tablets or drink 200 millilitres of a sugary beverage (juice, soft drink or similar). If possible, check blood glucose levels. Only get up once you feel back to normal, and the blood glucose levels have risen back to well above 80 milligrams per 100 millilitres (4.4 millimoles per litre).

CAUSES OF HYPOGLYCEMIA

Hypoglycemia can sometimes be caused by medications which increase the body's insulin production, and also by insulin treatment. The possible reasons for this include:

> More insulin than needed was injected by accident.

> There was too long a gap between medication intake/insulin injection and food intake.

> The meal's carbohydrate content was not high enough.

> More carbohydrates were consumed beforehand during additional activities.

> The insulin is working better due to weight loss.

> Larger quantities of alcohol impeded the body's production of glucose.

Advise your doctor if you experience hypoglycemia, particularly if this happens repeatedly and/or always at a similar time of day. Medication often needs to be adjusted in these cases.

TYPE 2 DIABETES
I STILL HAVE SOME QUESTIONS...

WHY IS THE NUMBER OF PEOPLE WITH TYPE 2 DIABETES GROWING?

When it comes to a cause, the answer lies around two important factors: diet and exercise. It is easy to give in to the convenience of processed foods. And since physical activity in everyday life is also drastically on the decline, more and more people are becoming overweight – which constitutes a significant risk factor.

CAN YOUNG PEOPLE ALSO BE AFFECTED BY WHAT IS COMMONLY KNOWN AS "ADULT-ONSET DIABETES"?

Yes, we no longer use the term "adult-onset diabetes", because people being diagnosed with type 2 diabetes in recent years have been getting increasingly younger due to the fact that children and young adults are becoming increasingly overweight. Sadly the "record" is currently held by a 7-year-old in Chicago weighing 222 kg (490 lbs).

WHY HAVE I DEVELOPED TYPE 2 DIABETES?

Insulin resistance is genetic. Whether this develops into diabetes depends on other factors, primarily excess weight and lack of exercise. Conversely, however, this also provides the opportunity to successfully treat type 2 diabetes with increased physical activity and a more health-conscious diet.

CAN I IDENTIFY THE RISK OF TYPE 2 DIABETES EARLY ON?

There is some important information to take into account with regards to the risk of developing type 2 diabetes: have your parents or grandparents had diabetes? Have you experienced one or more of the typical concomitant diseases such as excess weight, high blood pressure or lipometabolism disorders? The greater the number of applicable risk factors, the higher the risk of developing diabetes.

CAN I TAKE A TEST TO SEE WHETHER I AM GENETICALLY PREDISPOSED TO DEVELOPING TYPE 2 DIABETES?

The glucose tolerance test can provide information on this relatively early on. It shows whether intake of a specific quantity of glucose causes an abnormal rise in blood sugar levels. The oral glucose tolerance test (OGTT) is the most common type of test, though it is unnecessary if the fasting blood glucose levels are already abnormal.

WHEN IS GLUCOSE TOLERANCE CONSIDERED TO BE "IMPAIRED"?

Glucose tolerance can be considered impaired if blood sugar levels are still above 140 milligrams per 100 millilitres (7.8 millimoles per litre) two hours after the test has begun. Blood sugar levels over 200 milligrams per 100 millilitres (11.1 millimoles per litre) indicate the presence of diabetes mellitus.

WHAT IMPACT DO HIGH BLOOD GLUCOSE LEVELS HAVE ON EVERYDAY LIFE?

If the cells do not contain the sugar necessary for energy, then fatigue, exhaustion, skin changes, visual impairment and poor wound healing can significantly affect your general wellbeing. If you also have to urinate frequently at night, this can cause sleep disturbances and states of exhaustion, involving a lack of concentration and even depression.

CAN HIGH BLOOD GLUCOSE LEVELS CAUSE SERIOUS HEALTH PROBLEMS IN THE LONG-TERM?

Chronically elevated blood glucose levels are harmful to the small and large blood vessels. Typical complications include changes to the vessels in the fundus of the eyes, the kidneys and vascular walls. This in turn also affects the nervous system, leading to neuropathy involving dissociated sensations.

IS TYPE 2 DIABETES A LIFELONG DISEASE?

Insulin resistance does not go away. However, by normalising your weight and permanently changing your exercise and dietary habits, you can stop the insulin resistance from elevating your blood glucose levels. Ask your doctor whether medication should be taken for additional support.

LOSING WEIGHT
AND LIVING LIGHTER

IN MANY CASES, TYPE 2 DIABETES is associated with one or more other metabolic disorders including excess weight, high blood pressure, elevated blood lipids and HDL cholesterol deficiency. When these metabolic disorders occur collectively, the condition is known as "metabolic syndrome". Losing weight is the single most important way to counter these important risk factors.

LOSING WEIGHT EFFECTIVELY AND PERMANENTLY

In order to reduce body weight, there must be a negative energy balance, meaning that energy (food) intake must be less than the energy expended every day. Two approaches can be adopted to achieve this: firstly, you can increase your metabolic rate by exercising more every day and thus increasing physical activity. Secondly, you can limit your energy intake, meaning you can eat less and consume lower-calorie food. The best results are achieved when both approaches are combined.

EXERCISING MORE IN EVERYDAY LIFE

You don't need to put in peak performances to increase your metabolic rate. Exercising regularly is usually more than adequate.

Ideally you should also swim, walk or cycle for half an hour two to three times a week. These types of endurance sports are particularly beneficial as they protect the joints.

CALORIE BURN RATE FOR 15 MINUTES OF PHYSICAL ACTIVITY

Dancing	50 Cal
Bush walking	80 Cal
Walking	80 Cal
Playing golf	85 Cal
Cycling (15 km/h)	100 Cal
Swimming breaststroke	160 Cal
Running (11 km/h)	190 Cal

REDUCING ENERGY INTAKE – THE RIGHT WAY!

If you plan to eat less in order to lose weight, you should never do it in a drastic way, by only eating "half serves" of every meal or by skipping meals. If you do, you run the risk of not consuming enough carbohydrates to keep blood glucose levels constant.

The "eating half" method also reduces the intake of vitamins, minerals and other important nutrients which the body urgently needs to have in a balanced ratio, because it cannot produce them by itself.

This undersupply of nutrients and the stress on your metabolism that is associated with it can even delay the breakdown of body fat!

Reducing energy intake is only easy in the long run if the food is tasty and you can still eat until you feel full. This approach actually allows you to lose weight and protect yourself from the feared yo-yo effect where you lose weight and then put it straight back on again.

The recommended "diet" principle is less fancy, but

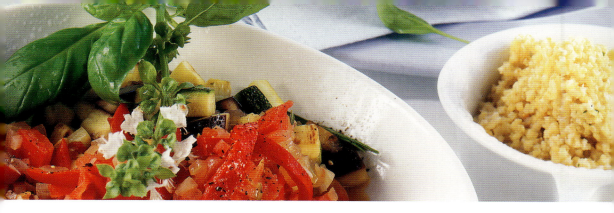

very effective: follow the most important rules of a balanced diet (see the box below) as well as the food pyramid recommendations (see the back cover flap). This will have a beneficial impact on your blood lipids and uric acid content as well.

All meals should predominantly comprise sufficient quantities of low-fat, vegetarian foods – wheat products, vegetables, potatoes and fruit – with smaller serves of animal products and meats, as well as valuable oils. Rapeseed oil and olive oil are particularly recommended. You don't have to abstain from eating sweets or drinking alcohol completely, but rather consume these in smaller quantities every so often.

To ensure that you continue to enjoy what you eat, we suggest you choose varied foods and prepare them in a tasty and, most importantly, healthy way.

THE MOST IMPORTANT TIPS FOR A BALANCED DIET

> Drink lots of water (1.5 to 3 litres daily), non-sparkling (where possible) water, as well as unsweetened herbal or fruit tea.
> Eat wholemeal bread or bran flakes several times a day.
> To ensure stable blood glucose levels, meals should contain a sufficient amount of potatoes, rice, noodles or other carbohydrates.
> Eat five servings of fruit and vegetables a day.
> Enrich your diet with low-fat dairy products.
> You can eat cheese daily in sandwiches, but limit the cold meat fillings such as salami.
> Eat ocean fish at least once a week.
> Reduce intake of animal fats.
> Preferably only eat meat, poultry or processed meat products three times a week.
> Use small amounts of high-quality vegetable oils (e.g. rapeseed oil, olive oil or safflower oil) several times a day to prepare vegetables and salads.
> Keep extras such as sweets, ice cream, cake or alcohol to a minimum, consuming them only on special occasions.

CARBOHYDRATES – THE LOWDOWN

FOR CARBOHYDRATE EXCHANGES (CE)

"CARBOHYDRATES" IS THE GENERIC TERM for starches, sugars and even dietary fibres (see also back cover flap). Of these, starch and sugar are the only available carbohydrates which directly affect blood glucose levels, and type 2 diabetics in particular are advised to consume these carbohydrates evenly throughout the day in order to take the strain off the pancreas. There are a number of different carbohydrate conversion formulae and measuring units designed to make it easier for you to prepare your meals.

CARBOHYDRATE EXCHANGES

Carbohydrate exchanges are probably the best-known conversion units among diabetics, and they have their own conversion tables. Carbohydrate exchanges (CEs) do not refer to the weight of a particular food – a slice of bread, for example, may weigh 40 g (1½ oz) but contain only 15 g (½ oz) carbohydrate.

CE tables show the standard quantity of food which contains 15 g (½ oz) realisable carbohydrates. But what exactly does this value mean? A carbohydrate serving equivalent to 1 CE raises the blood glucose levels by around 30–50 mg. Sufficient insulin must be provided accordingly to allow the sugar to enter the cells. For diabetics who are being treated with insulin, the number of carbohydrate exchange units they consume is an important criterion when selecting the ideal dose of insulin.

SOME EXAMPLES

1 CE is contained in:
60 g (½ oz) cooked white rice
75 g (2¾ oz) cooked white pasta
1 small to medium potato
1 small bread roll, 1 slice white bread
2 slices garlic bread, 1 slice thin pizza
1 fruit scone, 1 small cinnamon donut
1 tbsp jam, 2 tsp honey
4 prunes, 4 dates, 2 tbsp raisins
1 orange, 1 peach, 3 plums, 16 cherries
½ rockmelon, 4 large figs, 20 grapes
1 small banana, 1 apple, 6 apricots
3 kiwi fruits, 2 mandarins, 1 nectarine
90 g (3 oz) tinned chickpeas
120 g (4 oz) cooked lentils
250 ml (8 fl oz/1 cup) milk
1 tub low-fat plain yoghurt (200 g/6½ oz)
100 g (3⅓ oz) low-fat custard
4 small scoops ice cream

If you distribute carbohydrate intake evenly throughout the day, having several small meals rather than one large meal, the pancreas is put under less strain and your personal performance curve remains stable. The adjacent table shows you examples of how carbohydrates can be consumed throughout the day. A substitute table helps you exchange one carbohydrate serving with another to ensure the CE quantities remain the same.

NOT ALL CARBOHYDRATES ARE ALIKE!

The CE information can also be of use to those diabetics who do not require insulin treatment, allowing them to quickly assess the carbohydrate content of foods. It makes it easier to estimate serving sizes, thus also facilitating a sufficient and evenly spread intake of carbohydrates in the long term.

Only foods containing starch or sugar are taken into account for these measurements, that is all products from the bread/cereals/side dishes, sweets/drinks, fruit, and milk/soured milk products groups. Vegetables only contain small amounts of starch and sugar and are not counted when they are present in a quantity of less than 200 g (6½ oz) per meal.

ONLY HALF A BANANA?

Statements on fruit consumption, such as "Since being diagnosed with diabetes, I have to count really carefully when I eat cherries – I'm only allowed 16, so I prefer to eat an apple and not have to count", or "It's no fun eating a main course because I can only have a single small potato", come up in almost every diabetes training course. These assumptions are based on a misunderstanding of the illustrated carbohydrate exchange charts, which always show the food servings equivalent to 1 CE: for example 1 small to medium potato or 16 cherries, in this case.

This often leads to the incorrect assumption that what is listed are the maximum "allowed" quantities, frequently also resulting in an unhealthy limitation of foods containing carbohydrates. This may lead to some quite unpleasant effects: hunger, bad temper or even an unhealthy deficiency of important vitamins, minerals, dietary fibre and bio-active plant compounds.

Foods not providing any realisable carbohydrates such as cheese and ham, are often consumed as snacks, which totally defeats the purpose of losing weight and improving metabolism!

CONSISTENCY COUNTS

Be brave and do eat foods containing carbohydrates! Adults have a daily carbohydrate conversion rate of 180 g (5¾ oz), corresponding to 12 CEs. If you don't ingest these carbohydrates with food, your body has to obtain them from other sources – and you'll only regret it later.

AN EVEN SUPPLY OF CARBOHYDRATES DURING THE DAY - AN EXAMPLE

Meal	CE portions	Example	CE
1st Breakfast	4 x cereals	2 slices bread	2.7
2nd Breakfast	1 x fruit 1 x milk product	1 CE fruit 250 g (8 oz) yoghurt	1.3
Lunch	5 x accompaniments	75 g (2¾ oz) rice (raw weight)	3.3
Afternoon	1 x fruit	1 CE fruit	0.7
Evening	6 x cereals	3 slices bread	4
Late meal	1 x fruit 1 x milk product	1 CE fruit 250 g (8 oz) yoghurt	1.3

GLYCEMIC INDEX AND GLYCEMIC LOAD

MORE INDEXES...

THE GLYCEMIC INDEX,

which is often called the GI, ranks carbohydrate-containing foods based on their effect on blood glucose levels after being eaten. This effect is then compared with that of 50 g (1⅔ oz) glucose. Glucose is given the reference value of 100, and the index is a rating given to foods between 0 and 100. This can be grouped into low, medium and high values (see box below). The GI values apply to single food items only. The index's effect on blood sugar can also be significantly reduced if certain foods are combined in a meal.

> The glycemic index is considered to be high when values are between 70 and 100. This group includes glucose (100), cornflakes (84) and honey (73).
>
> Foods such as wholemeal bread (69), household sugar (65) and orange juice (57) have a medium GI with values ranging between 56 and 70, while grapes (52) and bananas (52) are fruits relatively high in sugar, and are thus ranked at the upper end of the low glycemic index.
>
> All foods with GI values of under 55 are classified as having a low glycemic index. Pulses (27-33), breakfast cereals, skim milk (32) and fructose (23), for example, have very low glycemic values, and vegetables have virtually no effect on blood glucose levels.

IT'S ALL ABOUT QUANTITY

Many foods with a low glycemic index are wholefoods providing a high nutrient density. This means, they are at the same time rich in dietary fibres, vitamins, minerals and other healthy components. It seems advisable for everyone to incorporate lots of carbohydrate-containing foods with low glycemic index into their daily diet, whether they are type 2 diabetic or not.

However, you should still always keep an eye on how much you eat too: the greater the quantity of foods with a low glycemic index that you consume, the more drastic the rise in blood glucose levels will be. If, on the other hand, you only eat a small quantity of food with a high glycemic index, the effect on blood glucose levels is not as intense as the high glycemic index actually suggests.

It is therefore always a question of balance and you will need to keep the overall picture in mind.

> The glycemic load of a food ranks the effect of a specific serving size of that food on blood glucose levels. The formula is this: glycemic index/100 x grams of carbohydrates per serving.

THE GLYCEMIC LOAD

The glycemic load shows how blood glucose levels are affected by the carbohydrates in a specific serving size of a food with high or low glycemic index, making it more suitable for rating foods in everyday life.

Depending on the serving size, the glycemic load of various foods can therefore be almost identical, despite vast differences in the glycemic index of these foods. This is easier to understand when we look at the comparison of two different types of bread.

EFFECT OF SERVING SIZE

100 g (3⅓ oz) multigrain bread contains 43 g (1½ oz) carbohydrates. The glycemic index of multigrain bread is 45. The glycemic load is 45/100 x 43 = 19.

100 g (3⅓ oz) white bread contains 48 g (1⅔ oz) carbohydrates. One serving is only equal to 50 g (1⅔ oz) white bread (24 g/¾ oz of carbohydrates). The glycemic index of white bread is 70. The glycemic load is 70/100 x 24 = 17.

1 serving (43 g) multigrain bread thus has a glycemic load of 19, while this is only 17 for 1 serving (48 g) of white bread. If you eat 100 g (3⅓ oz) white bread, that is more than 2 servings, the glycemic load rises to 34. So be careful with the serving size.

PRACTICAL TIPS

Food which is "low GI" means that the carbohydrates from the food are absorbed into the blood very slowly. Without insulin treatment, foods containing these "slow carbohydrates" are always an advantage, and similarly so for treatments using fast-acting insulin – including set combinations with slow-acting insulin, because the hormone does not take effect immediately after injecting. Carbohydrates and insulin are thus absorbed into the blood at roughly the same time. Are you being treated with fast-acting insulin analogues? Then it may be beneficial to inject the insulin while eating or even after eating (instead of beforehand, as is usually the case) when having meals with a lower glycemic index. This is a surefire way to prevent hypoglycemia.

> To ensure stable blood glucose levels, it is advisable to eat the following servings from the various food groups throughout the day:
> - at least 15 servings of wholemeal bread, cereals or potatoes
> - 4 servings (about 100 Cal each) of a low-fat dairy product, e.g. 200 ml (7 fl oz/¾ cup) skimmed milk, 250 g (8 oz) pure yoghurt, 30 g (1 oz) cheese
> - 3 servings of vegetables (200 g/6½ oz each)
> - 2 servings of fresh fruit (50-150 g/1⅔-5 oz each, depending on type) or dried fruit (15-20 g/½ oz-⅔ oz each, depending on type) or 100 ml (3 fl oz/½ cup) of fruit juice with no added sugar
> - 1 serving of pulses (with a gross weight of 75 g/2¾ oz, about 1 CE), or 100 g (3⅓ oz) lean meat, poultry or fish, or 1 egg, or 30 g (1 oz) sausage

One serving of carbohydrate-containing foods such as bread, cereals, potatoes, fruit, juice and dairy products equals about 1 CE (see page 14).

In addition, drink at least 6 glasses (300 ml/10 fl oz/1¼ cups each) and 2 cups (150 ml/5 fl oz/¾ cup each) water, tea or other calorie-free beverages. Use 2 tbsp oil, butter or margarine, or 2 servings of nuts or almonds (15 g/½ oz each) per day. And as a small bonus (1 CE and 100–150 Cal each), you can indulge in 1 chocolate bar, or 1 small piece of cake, or 1 handful of salted nuts, or 1 small glass of beer or wine.

EVERYDAY EATING
WITHOUT THE WORRY

WHAT DO I HAVE TO THINK ABOUT WHEN CHANGING MY EATING HABITS?

The most important thing is that eating remains a pleasant, social experience for you while also being "healthier". Fortunately, dietary recommendations for diabetics have improved drastically in recent years – they no longer include diets with long lists of prohibited foods. A healthy meal follows the guidelines of a balanced, varied diet (see pages 20–21).

WHAT IS THE IDEAL NUMBER OF MEALS?

To place less strain on the pancreas and to keep blood glucose levels steady, it is a good idea to spread your carbohydrate intake over five or six meals throughout the day. We recommend giving preference to foods with low glycemic index or servings with low glycemic load. More small meals rather than fewer large ones is a good rule for everyone.

SHOULD I EAT BETWEEN MEALS?

The answer is most certainly "yes" – if you are being treated with fast-acting insulin as part of a set insulin combination to prevent hypoglycemia. For other people, eating between meals has a relieving effect on blood glucose levels because the carbohydrates can be distributed more evenly. Discuss with your diabetes advisor or doctor whether or not you should be snacking between meals.

DO I HAVE TO EAT DIFFERENTLY WHEN PLAYING SPORT?

Physical activity, including gardening and housework, uses more energy and as such improves insulin function. As a precaution, you should therefore eat 1 extra CE for every 30-minute sports session if you inject insulin or are being treated with medication which increases the body's insulin production. This prevents hypoglycemia.

IS IT TRUE THAT DIABETICS CAN NOW EAT SUGAR?

Sugar is primarily a source of "empty energy", regardless of whether it is in the form of glucose, household sugar, honey or other sweeteners. As long as sugar and sugary foods are consumed in small quantities, they are harmless, even for diabetics. But beware of the "hidden sugars" – aside from jams and confectionery, most pastries, drinks and ready-made products generally also contain a lot of sugar.

WHAT ARE SUGAR SUBSTITUTES?

Sugar substitutes such as fructose or sugar alcohols (sorbitol, isomalt, xylitol) provide just as much energy, but have a lower glycemic index than household sugar (sucrose), and have little effect on blood glucose levels. Their only health-related advantage (even for diabetics) compared to sucrose is the fact that they cause fewer cavities. If consumed in excess, they can cause diarrhoea.

WHAT ARE SWEETENERS?

Sweeteners such as saccharin, acesulfame-K and cyclamate do not contain any energy. They do not affect blood sugar levels, but they do influence taste buds. Over time, you will grow accustomed to the sickly sweet taste. Foods containing sweeteners are labelled as such or bear a so-called E-number (E950, E951, E952, E953, E954, E957, E959).

IS IT BENEFICIAL TO USE SPECIAL DIABETIC PRODUCTS?

These foods will have an additional label stating that they are designed "for special diabetic diets", giving the impression that you can eat or drink as much of them as you want. But household sugar has usually only been replaced with sugar substitutes, sweeteners or a combination of these, nothing else. So the answer is a resounding "no".

HOW CAN I RELIABLY ESTIMATE THE CARBOHYDRATE CONTENT OF BOILED PASTA?

With a bit of practice you can, since boiled pasta absorbs varying amounts of water. The values depend on the noodle type, the manufacturer and the cooking time (hard or soft). Ideally you should weigh out the different varieties unprocessed, boil them until they reach the desired firmness, and then reweigh them. Memorise the quantity using a volume of measurement, such as a spoonful, plateful or ladleful.

EATING AND DRINKING

STAYING NOURISHED THROUGHOUT THE DAY

BREAKFAST NUMBER ONE – THE START TO THE DAY

The liver's rapidly available energy stores are empty after the overnight "fasting time" and the first meal of the day gives you your first source of energy. Brain and nerve foods such as wholegrain cereals, muesli and wholemeal bread combined with skim milk products and cheese are ideal. These can be supplemented with fresh fruit and vegetables such as cucumber, capsicum and tomato. A colourful breakfast like this is a real pick-me-up, giving you a great energy boost, and the combination of foods has a low glycemic load.

BREAKFAST NUMBER TWO AND THE AFTERNOON SNACK

One serving of fruit is a good source of fat-free carbohydrates, and is therefore an ideal snack. Fruit provides energy for the brain and nerves, and you can bridge the gap until your next main meal without having a slump. If your stomach is sensitive and you do not tolerate fruit acids well, or you want to further reduce the glycemic load of fruit, you can also combine plain yoghurt with fresh seasonal fruits.

The afternoon snack also aims to counter a drop in blood glucose levels. Low-fat snacks containing carbohydrates are ideal, even in the afternoon, which is why they too can include fresh fruit on their own or combined with yoghurt. Biscuits and cakes however should only be eaten on rare occasions, especially if you want to lose weight. Try and make them the exception, rather than the rule.

LUNCH – HOT OR COLD

This meal can be a hot dish if you prefer, and should contain a large serving of boiled potatoes (if possible with skin on), brown rice or wholemeal pasta and a large serving of vegetables, preferably sautéed in a small amount of high-quality vegetable oil (rapeseed or olive oil). A smaller serving of fish or lean meat – prepared in a low-fat way wherever possible – is a good accompaniment, while topping it with melted cheese, grated Parmesan or a sprinkling of some other type of hard cheese is a great source of valuable protein. Fresh fruit makes for a perfect, healthy dessert to round off the meal.

Lunch can also be a bread-based meal if this fits in better with your daily routine. However, carbohydrates and ingredients rich in protein and fat should be combined in a similar ratio to that of a hot meal.

DINNER – HOT OR COLD

The final main meal of the day is designed to satisfy while still being light, so as not to affect your sleep. You can choose whether you'd rather have a hot or cold meal, based on your daily routine and personal preferences. The assumption that a hot meal in the evening makes you put on weight is completely false – it is simply a matter of the meal's content, not the temperature at which it is served. For example, a cold dinner of wholefoods may be based on wholemeal bread with cheese, ideally served with a large salad dressed in a vinaigrette containing a small amount of high-quality oil. Combinations of wholemeal bread and marinated vegetables roasted in a dash of oil (antipasti) and some fish are examples of wholefood dinners which are easy to digest and do not put a strain on the body.

SUPPER

This final small meal of the day shortens the time of the overnight fast and prevents night-time hypoglycemia. It is particularly beneficial to eat foods containing calcium, ideally yoghurt, possibly with fresh fruit added, or some raw food (especially vegetables).

EATING IN HOTELS, CANTEENS AND RESTAURANTS

If there is no buffet option available where you can choose the serving sizes yourself, other meals often do not comply with diabetic recommendations. Meat servings are usually larger, while vegetable and side servings are smaller than advisable for healthy meals. Also fats are often used too liberally in the preparation of foods. Be aware of this, and try to balance it out with the meals you prepare yourself.

In any case, you can try to be clever when choosing the dishes. Avoid fatty sides such as fries, and crumbed or fried meat or fish. Do not choose any salad dressings containing mayonnaise or cocktail sauce. Salads containing egg, tuna and cheese sometimes even supply you with more energy than a full main course. Low-fat alternatives are fish, salads with vinegar and oil dressing, bread as a side, while a small grilled steak with a baked potato and a mixed salad makes for a good option on another day.

COMMON (INCORRECT) NOTIONS ABOUT EATING WITH DIABETES

"If you do eat cake, make sure it's a cream cake or cheesecake – this has less of an effect on blood glucose levels."

"It's better to nibble on a piece of cheese or cold meat rather than fruit if you're hungry between meals." "Sour apples contain less sugar than sweet varieties." "You are only allowed to eat the amount of noodles generally found in soups." "It's better to eat crispbread rather than normal bread or bread rolls."

All of these statements are completely unfounded, and are based on the incorrect assumption that you can successfully reduce the blood's glucose content by limiting dietary carbohydrates. As your main organs rely on the provision of carbohydrates, the body is sometimes able to produce carbohydrates itself. This means the blood still contains glucose, even if no carbohydrates are ingested with food.

In diabetics, sugar from the blood is either not eliminated into the cells at all (type 1) or is only done so to an inadequate extent (type 2). Treatment must therefore either provide insulin or improve its function. In the case of type 2 diabetes, this means normalising body weight by having a negative energy balance, aided by increased physical activity. Cakes and cold meats are therefore not good alternatives! The food pyramid on the cover flap makes it easier to see which foods should be eaten in larger quantities and which foods in much smaller quantities or rarely if at all. These rules apply to anyone – whether you are diabetic or not.

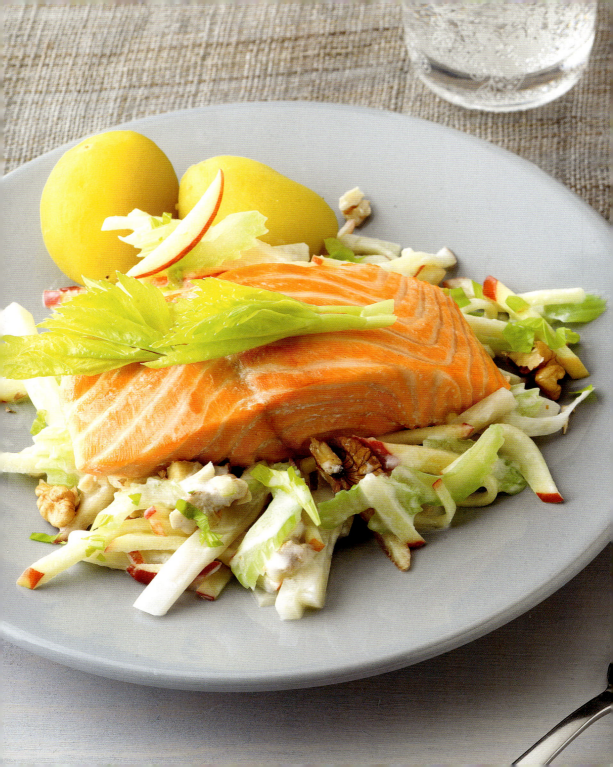

COOKING, BAKING AND ENJOYING

DIABETES-FRIENDLY GUARANTEED

Allow yourself to be seduced by the delicious recipes over the next few pages. All the dishes have been specially devised for a carbohydrate-conscious diet. They are simple to prepare and very tasty. The information on carbohydrate content and CE units is designed to make it easier for you to keep things in perspective. And depending on your individual needs, you can increase or reduce the quantity of carbohydrate-containing ingredients (cereals, pasta, rice).

Make your diet more varied, and therefore more enjoyable. The breakfast ideas, snacks and drinks, salads, soups and light meals, sweet treats and main courses in this book will soon convince you, your family and even your guests that a diabetic diet does not have to be any different from other dishes you would normally enjoy.

Muesli with fresh fruit

SERVES 2

5 tbsp mixed unsweetened wholegrain flakes

1 tsp sunflower seeds

3 tsp orange juice (alternatively apple juice)

400 g (13 oz) seasonal fruits (e.g. nectarines, plums, peaches, blackberries)

2 tsp lemon juice

200 g (6½ oz) cottage cheese

a few leaves of lemon balm or mint

PREPARATION: about 15 mins

1. In a non-stick pan lightly dry-roast the wholegrain flakes and the sunflower seeds without fat over medium heat, stirring constantly.
2. Transfer the flakes and the sunflower seeds to a bowl, stir in the juice and 50 ml (2 fl oz/¼ cup) water and leave to swell for about 5 minutes.
3. Meanwhile, depending on type of fruit used, wash, trim and chop into small pieces. Drizzle with the lemon juice. Gently fold the cottage cheese into the flake and seed mixture and transfer to plates or cereal bowls.
4. Arrange the fruit pieces on top. Garnish with a few lemon balm or mint leaves and serve.

TIP

Wholegrain cereal mixes usually contain wheat, barley, oat and spelt flakes. Unsweetened mixtures are generally available from health-food stores and from well-stocked chemists.

VARIATION

Peel and finely grate a piece of fresh ginger (about 2 cm/¾ in long). Stir the ginger into the cream cheese and sweeten to taste with 1–2 teaspoons apple or pear juice concentrate (from the healthfood store). Now fold into the cereal mix. If you do not have any fresh ginger, just use 1 pinch powdered ginger instead.

NUTRITIONAL VALUES PER PORTION:

315 Cal • 20 g protein • 8 g fat • 38 g carbohydrate • 8 g dietary fibre • about 2.4 CE

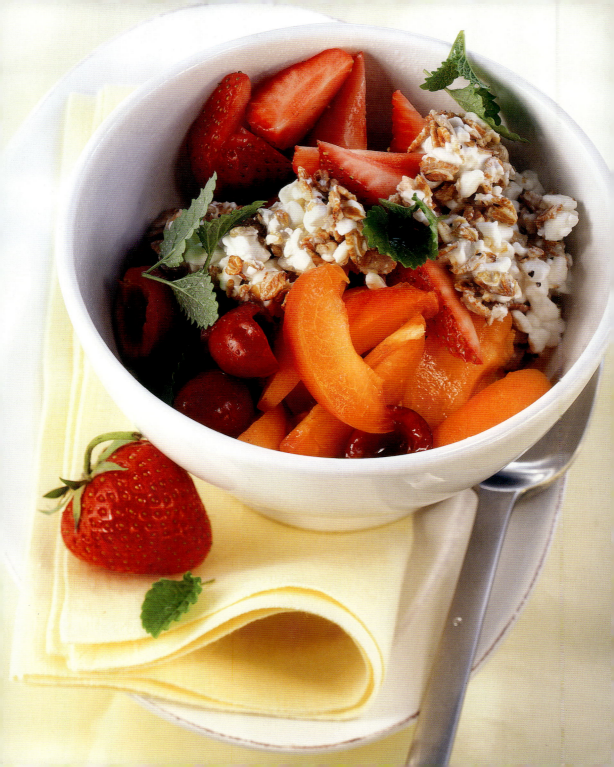

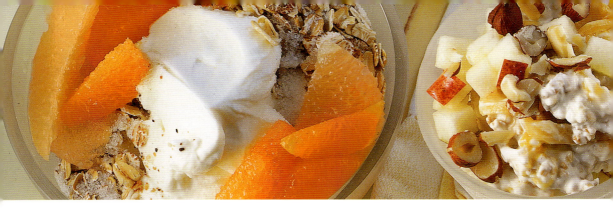

Citrus Fruit Muesli

SERVES 2

75 g (2¾ oz) crunchy wholemeal oat flakes
1 tsp sugar
2 seedless mandarins
1 pink grapefruit
200 g (6½ oz) cream cheese or yoghurt (0.2% fat)
liquid sweetener as desired

PREPARATION: about 15 mins

1. Briefly dry-roast the oat flakes in a non-stick pan without fat. Sprinkle over the sugar. Peel the mandarins and the grapefruit, divide into segments and cut into smaller pieces, reserving any juice.

2. Stir the citrus juice into the cream cheese until smooth. Flavour with sweetener to taste. Divide the cream cheese mixture between two bowls and cover with oat flakes and fruits.

NUTRITIONAL VALUES PER PORTION:

235 Cal • 13 g protein • 3 g fat • 40 g carbohydrate • 5 g dietary fibre • about 2.7 CE

Fresh Grain Muesli

SERVES 2

65 g (2¼ oz) wheat or oat grains
3 dried apricots
150 g (5 oz) low-fat yoghurt (1.5% fat)
1 large pear
1 tsp lemon juice
2 tbsp hazelnuts

PREPARATION: about 10 mins
SWELLING: 12 hrs

1. Roughly crack the grains in a cereal mill. Cut the apricots into strips. Stir 6 tablespoons water and 3 tablespoons yoghurt into the grains and apricots. Cover and leave to swell overnight in the fridge.

2. Wash and quarter the pear. Remove the core. Dice the pear quarters and drizzle with lemon juice. Chop the hazelnuts. Spread the remaining yoghurt, pear pieces and hazelnuts over the grain mixture.

NUTRITIONAL VALUES PER PORTION:

265 Cal • 9 g protein • 8 g fat • 39 g carbohydrate • 7 g dietary fibre • about 2.7 CE

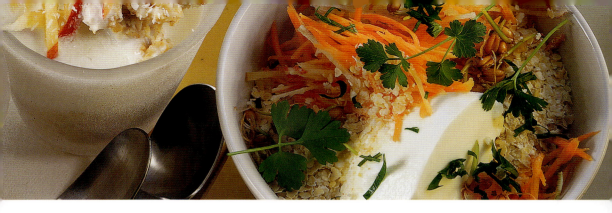

Apple & Coconut Porridge

SERVES 2
75 g (2¾ oz) cereal flakes
2 tbsp desiccated coconut
liquid sweetener as desired
2 small red apples
1 tsp lemon juice
180 g (5¾ oz) buttermilk
PREPARATION: about 10 mins

1. In a saucepan, bring to the boil the cereal flakes and coconut in 190 ml (7 fl oz/¾ cup) water, then leave to lightly simmer for 2 minutes. Sweeten as desired and arrange in bowls.

2. Wash, quarter and core the apples, cut the flesh into sticks and combine with the lemon juice. Arrange on top of the porridge and pour over the buttermilk.

NUTRITIONAL VALUES PER PORTION:
300 Cal • 8 g protein • 11 g fat • 40 g carbohydrate • 8 g dietary fibre • about 2.7 CE

Hearty Millet Muesli

SERVES 2
5 tbsp millet flakes
1 tbsp wheatgerm
250 g (8 oz) sour milk
1 tbsp chopped parsley
1 large apple (about 180 g/5¾ oz)
2 carrots
2 tsp lemon juice
PREPARATION: about 10 mins

1. Stir together the millet flakes, wheatgerm, 150 g (5 oz) sour milk and parsley. Wash, quarter and core the apple; peel the carrots. Roughly grate the apple and the carrots and drizzle with the lemon juice.

2. Stir about half the grated apple and carrot into the millet mixture, then divide the remaining sour milk, apple and carrot over the top.

NUTRITIONAL VALUES PER PORTION:
210 Cal • 9 g protein • 2 g fat • 40 g carbohydrate • 7 g dietary fibre • about 2.7 CE

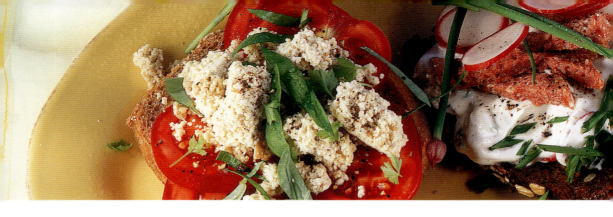

Bread Roll with basil tofu

SERVES 2

100 g (3⅓ oz) smoked tofu
2 tbsp freshly chopped basil (or parsley)
salt, pepper
3 small tomatoes
2 wholemeal rye bread rolls (50 g/1⅔ oz)
basil leaves, extra

PREPARATION: about 10 mins

1. Mash the tofu with a fork or briefly purée in a food processor or using a hand-held blender. Stir in the basil. Season the mixture with salt and pepper to taste. Wash the tomatoes and cut into thin slices.

2. Cut the bread rolls in half and cover each half with tomato slices. Spread the basil tofu on top and serve with some extra basil leaves.

NUTRITIONAL VALUES PER PORTION:
245 Cal • 10 g protein • 4 g fat • 42 g carbohydrate • 4 g dietary fibre • about 2.7 CE

Corned Beef Open Sandwich

SERVES 2

6 radishes
2 tbsp low-fat cream cheese
1 tbsp snipped chives
salt, pepper
2 slices wholemeal bread (55 g/2 oz)
100 g (3⅓ oz) corned beef

PREPARATION: about 15 mins

1. Wash and trim the radishes, then cut into thin slices. Set some aside for garnishing. Stir a little water into the cream cheese until smooth. Stir in the radish slices and ½ tablespoon chives. Season with salt and pepper, and spread the bread with the mixture.

2. Cut the corned beef into strips or dice and spread these on top of the radish cream cheese. Sprinkle with the remaining chives and some radish slices and serve.

NUTRITIONAL VALUES PER PORTION:
260 Cal • 19 g protein • 3 g fat • 36 g carbohydrate • 6 g dietary fibre • about 2.4 CE

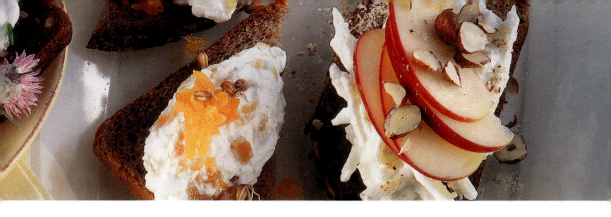

Cheese & Apricot Open Sandwich

SERVES 2

200 g (6½ oz) cottage cheese
liquid sweetener as desired
50 g (1⅔ oz) soft dried apricots
2 slices wholemeal bread
  (60 g/2 oz)
2 tsp wheatgerm

PREPARATION: about 10 mins

1. Sweeten the cottage cheese to taste. Finely chop the apricots, reserve 1 teaspoon and combine the rest with the cottage cheese.

2. Cut the bread slices diagonally so you have four triangles. Using two moistened tablespoons, take dollops of the cheese mixture and place on the bread triangles. Sprinkle with the remaining apricots and the wheatgerm.

NUTRITIONAL VALUES PER PORTION:
280 Cal • 23 g protein • 3 g fat • 36 g carbohydrate • 7 g dietary fibre • 2.4 CE

Apple & Cream Cheese Open Sandwich

SERVES 2

1 apple
1 tsp lemon juice
100 g (3⅓ oz) low-fat cream cheese
2 tbsp chopped hazelnuts
2 slices wholemeal bread
  (60 g/2 oz)

PREPARATION: about 10 mins

1. Wash, quarter and core the apple, then roughly grate three of the quarters. Cut the remaining quarter into thin wedges. Drizzle everything with lemon juice.

2. Stir a little water into the cream cheese until smooth. Stir in the grated apple and the hazelnuts, reserving some for garnishing. Spread the bread with the cream cheese mixture and garnish with the apple wedges and some hazelnuts.

NUTRITIONAL VALUES PER PORTION:
270 Cal • 11 g protein • 6 g fat • 40 g carbohydrate • 6 g dietary fibre • about 2.7 CE

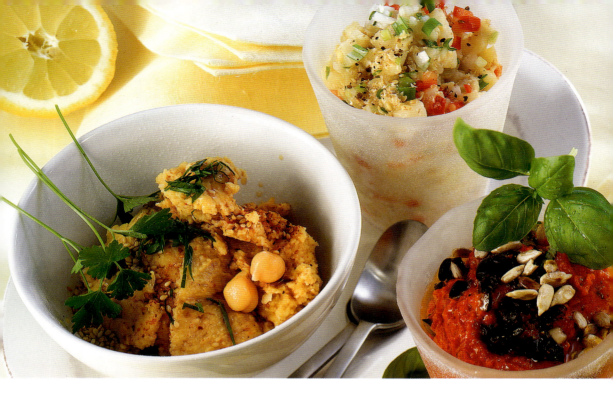

Hummus with sesame seeds

SERVES 2
1 tbsp unhulled sesame seeds
1 small tin chickpeas (drained weight 125 g/4 oz)
½ tsp lemon juice
salt
1 tsp chopped parsley
1 tsp sesame oil
1 pinch cayenne pepper
PREPARATION: about 10 mins

1. Dry-roast the sesame seeds in a non-stick pan without fat, then leave to cool. Purée the chickpeas and season them with the lemon juice and a little salt.
2. Stir in the parsley, the sesame seeds and the sesame oil. Flavour the hummus with cayenne pepper to taste.

SERVE WITH BREAD
Adjust the amount according to your daily carbohydrate requirements: ½ slice bread or ½ bread roll (about 25 g/¾ oz each) supply 0.7 CE.

TIP
Why not make double the amount of hummus? Put the spread in a screw-top jar and cover it with sesame oil; that way it will keep for about 3 days in the fridge.

NUTRITIONAL VALUES PER PORTION:
155 Cal • 7 g protein • 8 g fat • 13 g carbohydrate • 7 g dietary fibre • about 0.7 CE

Eggplant Spread with capsicum

SERVES 2

200 g (6½ oz) eggplant (aubergine)
3 tsp olive oil
1 spring onion
½ small red capsicum (pepper)
1 tsp lemon juice
1 small garlic clove
2 tsp oat bran
salt, pepper

PREPARATION: about 25 mins

1. Wash and trim the eggplant, thinly peel, then cut the flesh into small dice. Brush a non-stick pan with 1 teaspoon oil, add the eggplant, cover and sauté over medium heat for about 15 minutes until soft, turning a few times.

2. Meanwhile trim and wash the spring onion, then cut into thin rings. Trim, wash and finely chop the capsicum half. Using a fork, roughly mash the eggplant and drizzle it with the lemon juice. Peel and crush the garlic, then add to the mixture. Stir in the spring onion, capsicum and oat bran. Season the eggplant spread with salt and pepper.

SERVE WITH BREAD

Adjust the amount according to your daily carbohydrate requirements: ½ slice bread or ½ bread roll (about 25 g/¾ oz each) supply 0.7 CE.

NUTRITIONAL VALUES PER PORTION:
110 Cal • 2 g protein • 7 g fat • 7 g carbohydrate • 4 g dietary fibre • about 0.7/1.3 CE

Olive & Roasted Vegetable Paste

SERVES 2

6 pitted black olives
2 sprigs basil
1 tsp sunflower seeds
4 tbsp ajvar (relish from the jar, 80 g/2¾ oz)
1 tsp olive oil
pepper

PREPARATION: about 10 mins

1. Finely dice the olives. Wash and shake dry the basil, then cut the leaves into fine strips. Chop the sunflower seeds.

2. Combine the olives, basil and sunflower seeds with the ajvar. Add the oil and stir well. Season to taste with pepper.

SERVE WITH BREAD

Adjust the amount according to your daily carbohydrate requirements: ½ slice bread or ½ bread roll (about 25 g/¾ oz each) supply 0.7 CE.

VARIATION

The spread will be more filling if you add 20 g (²/₃ oz) finely chopped sheep's cheese into the mixture.

NUTRITIONAL VALUES PER PORTION:
60 Cal • 1 g protein • 5 g fat • 3 g carbohydrate • 1 g dietary fibre • 0 CE

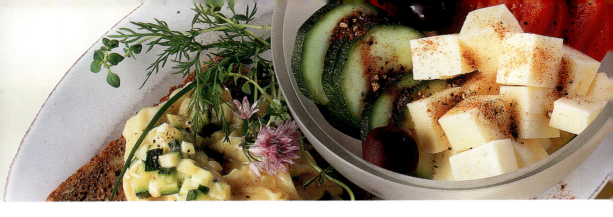

Zucchini Scrambled Eggs

SERVES 2

150 g (5 oz) zucchini (courgette)
2 tsp rapeseed oil
3 eggs
2 tbsp mineral water
salt, pepper
2 tbsp chopped mixed herbs
2 slices wholemeal bread (about 60 g/2 oz)

PREPARATION: about 15 mins

1. Wash, trim and finely chop the zucchini. Heat the oil in a non-stick frying pan, add the zucchini pieces and sauté for about 2 minutes.

2. Whisk the eggs with the mineral water, salt, pepper and the herbs. Pour over the zucchini and fry over low heat until set.

> **SERVE WITH BREAD**
> Adjust the amount according to your daily carbohydrate requirements: ½ slice bread or ½ bread roll (about 25 g/¾ oz each) supply 0.7 CE.

NUTRITIONAL VALUES PER PORTION:
380 Cal • 19 g protein • 15 g fat • 40 g carbohydrate • 7 g dietary fibre • about 2.7 CE

Cheese & Vegetable Snack

SERVES 2

200 g (6½ oz) cucumber
4 small tomatoes
100 g (3⅓ oz) piece of low-fat semi-hard cheese (e.g. Edam or Cheddar, 30% fat)
6 stoned black olives
salt, pepper
1 large pinch sweet paprika

PREPARATION: about 10 mins

1. Wash and thinly slice the cucumber and the tomatoes. Dice the cheese.

2. Arrange the cucumber and tomato slices, the cheese dice and the olives on serving plates or in bowls. Season to taste with salt, pepper and paprika.

> **SERVE WITH BREAD**
> Adjust the amount according to your daily carbohydrate requirements: ½ slice bread or ½ bread roll (about 25 g/¾ oz each) supply 0.7 CE.

NUTRITIONAL VALUES PER PORTION:
155 Cal • 14 g protein • 10 g fat • 3 g carbohydrate • 1 g dietary fibre • 0 CE

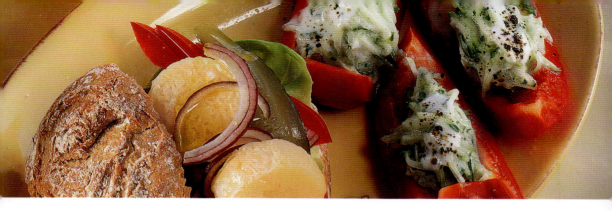

Cheese & Salad Rolls

SERVES 2

4 lettuce leaves
1 small red capsicum (pepper)
1 red onion, 1 gherkin
100 g (3⅓ oz) Harzer cheese (or haloumi)
2 wholemeal rye bread rolls (50 g/1⅔ oz)
2 tsp oil, 1 tsp white vinegar

PREPARATION: about 10 mins

1. Wash and shake dry the lettuce leaves. Trim and wash the capsicum; cut into strips. Peel the onion and cut into thin rings; slice the gherkin lengthways. Cut the cheese into slices. If using haloumi, lightly fry for a few minutes on each side.

2. Halve the rolls. On each bottom half arrange the lettuce, capsicum strips, onion rings gherkin slices and cheese. Stir together the oil and the white vinegar and drizzle over the top. Cover with the top halves of the rolls and serve.

NUTRITIONAL VALUES PER PORTION:
300 Cal • 22 g protein • 7 g fat • 42 g carbohydrate • 7 g dietary fibre • about 2.7 CE

Capsicum Boats with tzatziki

SERVES 2

150 g (5 oz) cucumber
150 g (5 oz) yoghurt (3.5% fat)
1 tsp white wine vinegar
1 tsp olive oil
salt, pepper
1 small red capsicum (pepper)

PREPARATION: about 15 mins

1. Wash and trim the cucumber. Halve lengthways, scrape out the seeds. Grate the flesh. Stir it into the yoghurt. Season with vinegar, oil, salt and pepper.

2. Halve, trim and wash the capsicum. Cut each half into thirds lengthways. Place the cucumber yoghurt into the boats.

> **SERVE WITH BREAD**
> Adjust the amount according to your daily carbohydrate requirements:
> ½ slice bread or ½ bread roll (about 25 g/¾ oz each) supply 0.7 CE.

NUTRITIONAL VALUES PER PORTION:
90 Cal • 4 g protein • 5 g fat • 6 g carbohydrate • 3 g dietary fibre • about 0.5 CE

Ham Rolls with radishes

SERVES 2

250 g (8 oz) large white radish
salt
1 spring onion
4 small radishes
1 tbsp pumpkin seed oil (or rapeseed oil)
1 tbsp yoghurt (3.5% fat)
1 tbsp lemon juice
pepper
2 heaped tsp pumpkin seeds
2 wholemeal multigrain bread rolls (50 g/1⅔ oz)
1 tsp margarine
1 tsp Dijon mustard
4 thin slices ham (40 g/1½ oz)

PREPARATION: about 15 mins

1. Wash, trim and thinly peel the large radish, then grate medium fine. Sprinkle with salt and leave for 5 minutes to draw out the moisture. Wash and trim the spring onion; finely chop. Wash and trim the radishes.

2. Whisk the oil, yoghurt and lemon juice together to make a dressing. Season with pepper. Combine the radish and spring onion and add the dressing. Dry-roast the pumpkin seeds in a non-stick pan without fat, then roughly chop.

3. Halve the rolls. Spread with margarine and mustard and cover with the ham. Sprinkle the pumpkin seeds on top of the chopped radish and serve with the ham rolls. Garnish with the small whole radishes.

TIP

Stir ¼ teaspoon finely grated ginger into the salad dressing – it will make the radish much easier to digest.

NUTRITIONAL VALUES PER PORTION:
360 Cal • 12 g protein • 16 g fat • 40 g carbohydrate • 6 g dietary fibre • about 2.7 CE

Herring Salad on wholegrain bread

SERVES 2

3 gherkins
½ apple
1 tsp lemon juice
1 small carrot
75 g (2¾ oz) fresh beetroot
3 sprigs dill
1 small red (Spanish) onion
2 Swedish pickled herring fillets (in a sweet and sour marinade, about 125 g/4 oz)
1 tbsp yoghurt salad cream (11% fat)
pepper
4 lettuce leaves (e.g. butter)
2 slices wholemeal bread (60 g/2 oz)

PREPARATION: about 15 mins

1. Finely chop the gherkins. Wash, halve and core the apple, then finely dice and drizzle with the lemon juice. Cut the carrot and beetroot into thin strips.

2. Wash and shake dry the dill, then chop, leaving a few sprigs for garnishing. Peel and chop the onion. Dice the herring fillets. Transfer the herring, gherkin, apple and vegetable strips to a bowl. Add the dill, onion and salad cream. Season with pepper to taste and stir well until all combined.

3. Wash and shake dry the lettuce leaves. Halve the bread slices and cover each half with a lettuce leaf. Arrange the herring salad on top and garnish with the reserved dill tips.

VARIATION

For a change, make this salad with smoked salmon instead of the pickled herring.

NUTRITIONAL VALUES PER PORTION:
375 Cal • 16 g protein • 17 g fat • 37 g carbohydrate • 7 g dietary fibre • 2.4 CE

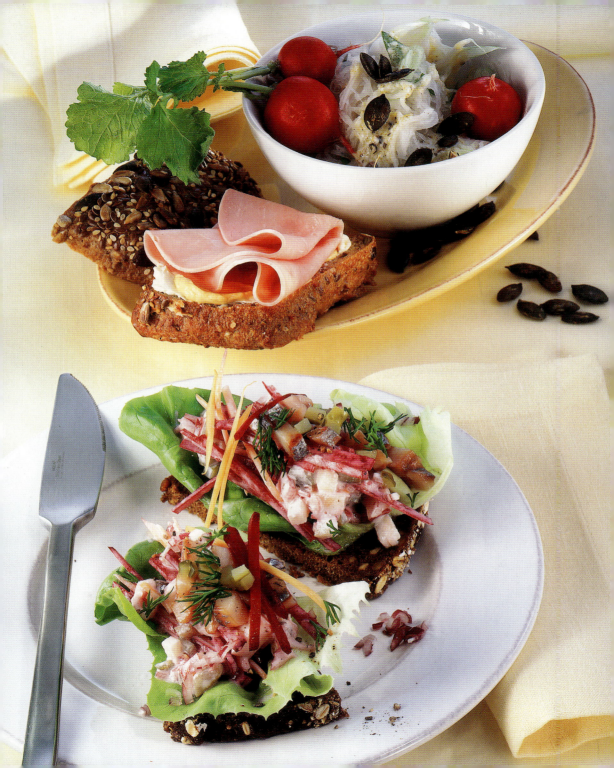

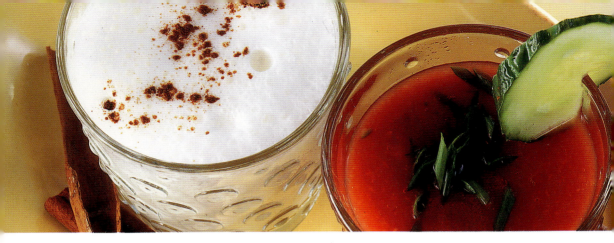

Indian Lassi

MAKES 2 GLASSES

150 g (5 oz) low-fat yoghurt (1.5% fat)
2 tbsp sour cream (10% fat)
1 pinch ground cardamom
1 pinch ground cinnamon
liquid sweetener as desired

PREPARATION: about 5 mins

1. Using a food processor or a hand-held blender whisk the yoghurt with the sour cream, cardamom, cinnamon and 100 ml (3 fl oz/½ cup) water until the mixture is foamy.

2. Flavour the yoghurt shake with liquid sweetener to taste and serve in tall glasses.

TIP
You don't fancy yoghurt? Just replace with buttermilk, sour cream or a soy-based drink instead.

NUTRITIONAL VALUES PER PORTION:
50 Cal • 3 g protein • 3 g fat • 4 g carbohydrate • 0 g dietary fibre • 0 CE

Vegetable Drink

MAKES 2 GLASSES

150 g (5 oz) cucumber
300 ml (10 fl oz/1¼ cup) red vegetable juice
sweet paprika
2 tbsp snipped chives

PREPARATION: about 10 mins

1. Peel the cucumber. Cut off 2 thin slices and set aside. Cut the remaining cucumber into small pieces and finely purée together with the vegetable juice using a food processor or a hand-held blender.

2. Season the vegetable drink with sweet paprika and pour into tall glasses. Cut the reserved cucumber slices almost in half and stick on the side of the glass. Sprinkle with snipped chives and serve.

NUTRITIONAL VALUES PER PORTION:
20 Cal • 1 g protein • 0 g fat • 4 g carbohydrate • 0 g dietary fibre • 0 CE

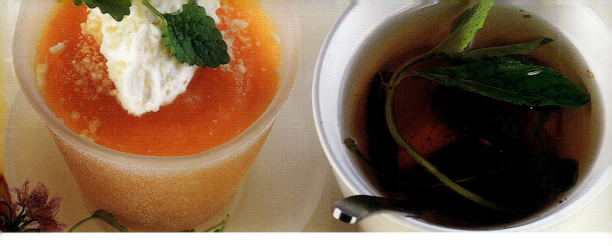

Peach frappé with cream

MAKES 2 GLASSES

700 g (1 lb 6 oz) ripe, chilled peaches
4 tbsp lime juice (or lemon juice)
4 tbsp cream
liquid sweetener as desired
2 tsp finely chopped almonds
a few leaves lemon balm or mint
PREPARATION: about 15 mins

1. Briefly dip the peaches into boiling water, then remove, rinse under cold water and slip off the skins. Halve the fruits, remove the stones and finely purée the flesh with the lime or lemon juice in a food processor or using a hand-held blender. Pour into two tall glasses.

2. Whisk the cream with sweetener as desired (using a milk foamer if you have one). Fold in the almonds. Place a dollop of the cream on the fruit purée and garnish with lemon balm or mint.

NUTRITIONAL VALUES PER PORTION:

225 Cal • 3 g protein • 12 g fat • 23 g carbohydrate • 5 g dietary fibre • about 1.3 CE

Vanilla & Ginger Tea

MAKES 4 GLASSES

30 g (1 oz) fresh ginger
½ vanilla pod
300 ml (10 fl oz/1¼ cup) clear apple juice
4 sprigs mint (or spearmint)
PREPARATION: about 20 mins

1. Peel and finely slice the ginger. Split the vanilla pod lengthways. Place both in a saucepan with 400 ml (14 fl oz/1¾ cups) water, bring to the boil, cover and simmer for 15 minutes. Add the apple juice.

2. Wash the mint and place one sprig into each mug or glass. Strain the tea and pour into each mug or glass. Serve hot or chilled.

NUTRITIONAL VALUES PER PORTION:

45 Cal • 0 g protein • 0 g fat • 10 g carbohydrate • 0 g dietary fibre • about 0.7 CE

Bean Salad with tuna

SERVES 2

300 g (10 oz) snowpeas (mange tout)

salt

1 handful celery leaves

1 small tin kidney beans (drained weight 125 g/4 oz)

1 tin tuna in brine (drained weight 150 g/5 oz)

½ small red (Spanish) onion

pepper

½ tsp Dijon mustard

2 tbsp red wine vinegar

2 tbsp olive oil

4 lettuce leaves

6 cherry tomatoes

PREPARATION: about 25 mins
MARINATING: about 15 mins

1. Wash, trim and halve the beans. In a saucepan, bring salted water to the boil. Add half the celery leaves and the beans. Cook over medium heat for about 2 minutes until firm to the bite. Drain the beans and rinse under cold water, then leave to drain well again.

2. Drain the kidney beans, rinse under cold water and drain again. Drain the tuna, reserving the brine. Flake the tuna with a fork.

3. Wash and shake dry the remaining celery leaves. Finely chop the leaves. Peel and dice the onion.

4. Whisk together the chopped celery leaves with the salt, pepper, mustard, vinegar and 1 tablespoon tuna brine. Stir in the oil. Combine the beans with the onions and tuna and pour over the dressing. Cover the salad and leave to marinate for at least 15 minutes.

5. Wash and shake dry the lettuce leaves. Wash the tomatoes and cut into eighths. Line two small salad bowls with the lettuce leaves. Combine the tomatoes with the bean salad. Season to taste with salt and pepper. Arrange the salad in two bowls on top of the lettuce.

SERVE WITH BREAD
Adjust the amount according to your daily carbohydrate requirements: ½ slice bread or ½ bread roll (about 25 g/¾ oz each) supply 0.7 CE.

TIP
When in season, this salad is just as tasty with French beans, yellow butter beans or any other green beans. Instead of fresh beans you can also use frozen ones.

NUTRITIONAL VALUES PER PORTION:
270 Cal • 20 g protein • 12 g fat • 20 g carbohydrate • 3 g dietary fibre • about 1.3 CE

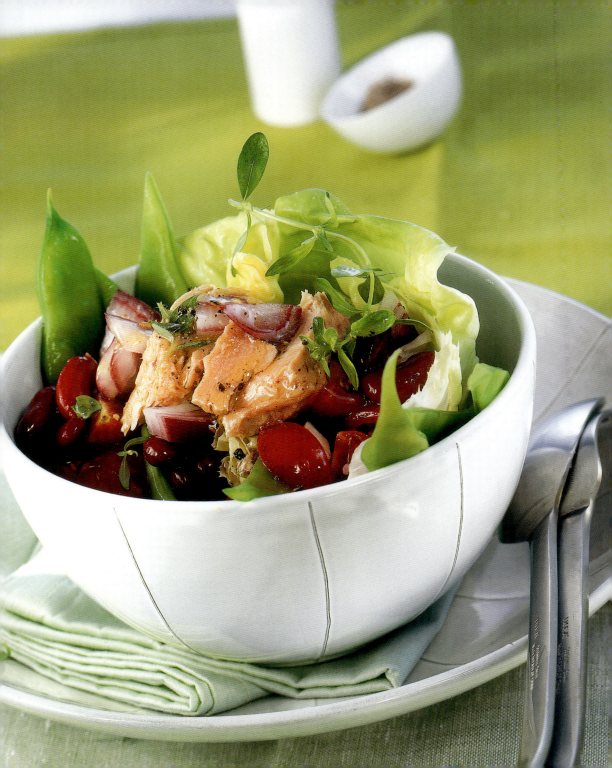

Chicory & Grape Salad with cheese dressing

SERVES 2

2 chicory heads (350 g/11½ oz)
200 g (6½ oz) small red grapes
80 g (2¾ oz) herbed cream cheese (30% fat)
1 tsp tomato paste
4-5 tbsp low-fat milk (1.5% fat)
salt, pepper

PREPARATION: about 20 mins

1. Trim the chicory, cutting out the bitter core in a wedge shape. Separate the individual leaves, wash and drain well. Cut the lower halves of the leaves into thin strips. Wash, halve and deseed the grapes if necessary.

2. To make the salad dressing, mash the cream cheese with a fork, then stir in the tomato paste and 4–5 tablespoons milk. Season with salt and pepper.

3. Arrange the tops of the chicory leaves in a circle on two serving plates or bowls. Put the chicory strips into the centre of each serving and drizzle with the dressing. Arrange the grape halves evenly on top.

> **TIP**
> Chicory is available with either yellow or red leaves. This specialist vegetable has a distinctive bitter flavour. If you are not using it immediately, it is best stored in the fridge.

> **SERVE WITH BREAD**
> Adjust the amount according to your daily carbohydrate requirements:
> ½ slice bread or ½ bread roll (about 25 g/¾ oz each) supply 0.7 CE.

NUTRITIONAL VALUES PER PORTION:
150 Cal • 9 g protein • 4 g fat • 22 g carbohydrate • 2 g dietary fibre • about 1.3 CE

Warm Savoy Cabbage Salad

SERVES 2

400 g (13 oz) young savoy cabbage
1 small red capsicum (pepper)
4 tbsp orange juice
3 tbsp white wine vinegar
salt, pepper
½ tsp mustard
1 tbsp olive oil

PREPARATION: about 20 mins

1. Remove the coarse outer leaves from the cabbage. Separate the remaining leaves, wash and cut out the central stems. Cut the leaves into thin strips and blanch these in boiling salted water for about 3 minutes. Drain, rinse under cold water and leave to drain.

2. Trim, quarter and wash the capsicum. Cut the flesh into very fine strips.

3. Whisk the orange juice with 2 tablespoons vinegar, salt, pepper, mustard and oil to make a dressing. Season to taste with the remaining vinegar.

4. Combine the warm cabbage with the capsicum strips and the dressing. Season to taste with salt and pepper and serve lukewarm.

> **SERVE WITH BREAD**
> Adjust the amount according to your daily carbohydrate requirements:
> ½ slice bread or ½ bread roll (about 25 g/¾ oz each) supply 0.7 CE.

NUTRITIONAL VALUES PER PORTION:
115 Cal • 6 g protein • 6 g fat • 10 g carbohydrate • 6 g dietary fibre • about 0.7 CE

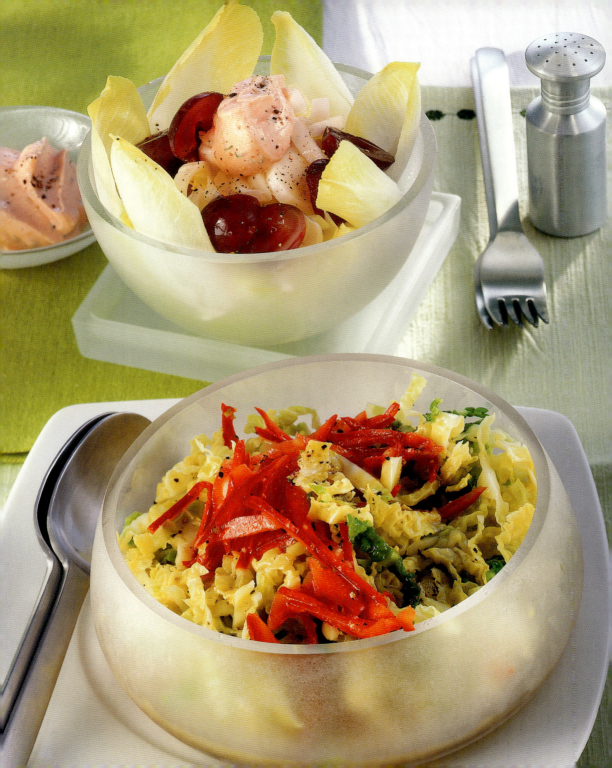

Chickpea Salad with herb dressing

SERVES 2

1 tin chickpeas (250 g/8 oz drained weight)
250 g (8 oz) cherry tomatoes
2 spring onions
1 sprig mint (or basil)
½ bunch flat-leaf parsley
150 g (5 oz) yoghurt (3.5% fat)
2 tbsp lemon juice
grated zest of ¼ organic lemon
1 small garlic clove
1 tbsp olive oil
salt, pepper
1 large pinch ground cumin (or ground allspice)
1 large pinch cayenne pepper

PREPARATION: about 20 mins
MARINATING: about 30 mins

1. Drain the chickpeas, rinse under cold water and leave to drain. Wash the tomatoes. Trim, wash and finely chop the spring onions.

2. Wash and shake dry the mint and the parsley. Pull off the leaves and chop finely. Using a food processor or hand-held blender purée the herbs, yoghurt, lemon juice and zest, until you have a light green dressing. Peel then crush the garlic and add to the dressing. Stir in the oil. Season with salt, pepper, cumin and cayenne pepper to taste.

3. Put the chickpeas, tomatoes and spring onions into a bowl. Pour over the herb dressing and gently stir to combine. Cover the chickpea salad and leave to stand at room temperature for 30 minutes to draw flavour before serving.

NUTRITIONAL VALUES PER PORTION:
295 Cal • 16 g protein • 10 g fat • 35 g carbohydrate • 15 g dietary fibre • 2.3 CE

Couscous Salad

SERVES 2

200 g (6½ oz) carrots
200 ml (7 fl oz/¾ cup) vegetable stock
100 g (3⅓ oz) couscous
1½ tbsp olive oil
5 tbsp lemon juice
salt, pepper
2 spring onions
250 g (6½ oz) tomatoes
½ bunch dill

PREPARATION: about 20 mins

1. Trim, peel the carrots and cut into small pieces. Simmer in the stock for 2 minutes. Put the couscous into a bowl, then pour over the hot stock including the carrots. Stir in the oil and 3 tablespoons lemon juice. Season the couscous with salt and pepper and leave to expand for about 10 minutes.

2. Meanwhile, trim, wash and thinly slice the spring onions. Wash and finely chop the tomatoes. Wash and shake dry the dill, set aside a few sprigs for the garnishing and finely chop the rest.

3. Fluff the couscous with a fork. Fold in the spring onions, tomatoes and dill. Season the salad with salt and pepper and add the remaining lemon juice to taste. Garnish the salad with the remaining dill and serve.

TIP
Couscous is available from all good supermarkets and delis. Instant couscous does not have to be cooked again, simply leave the grains to swell as per packet instructions.

NUTRITIONAL VALUES PER PORTION:
300 Cal • 8 g protein • 10 g fat • 44 g carbohydrate • 9 g dietary fibre • about 2.7 CE

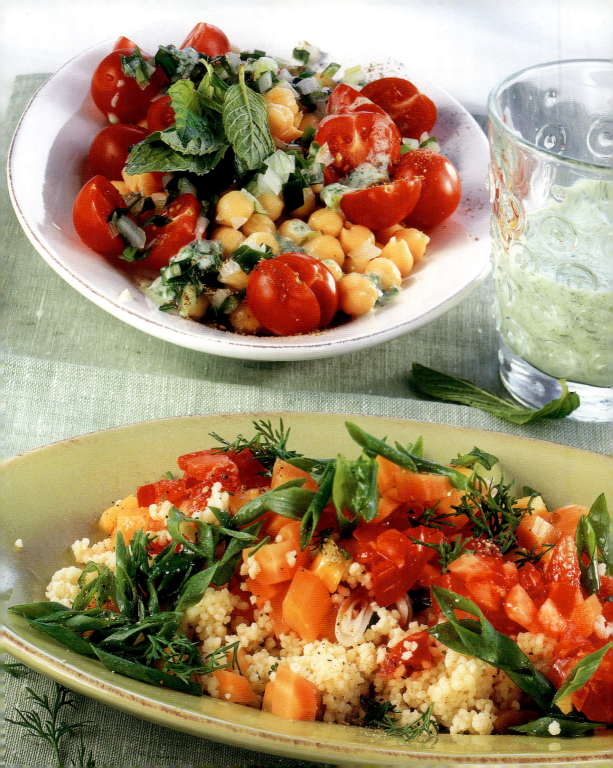

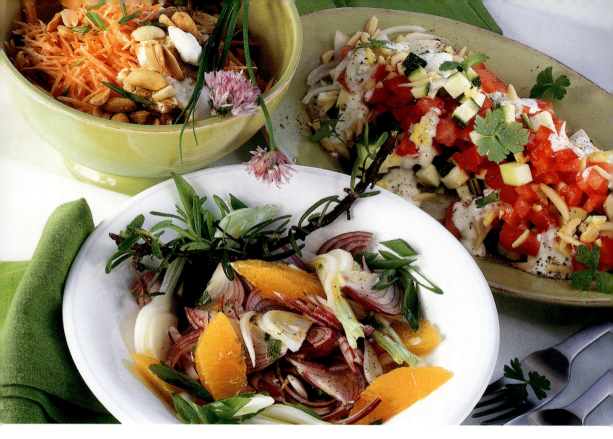

Moroccan Carrot Salad

SERVES 2

1 tbsp rapeseed oil
½ tsp ground cardamom
½ tsp ground ginger
4 tbsp buttermilk
300 g (10 oz) carrots
1 tbsp roasted unsalted peanuts
salt
1 tbsp snipped chives
PREPARATION: about 20 mins

1. Heat the oil in a frying pan. Add the cardamom and the ginger and fry briefly. Remove from the heat and stir into the buttermilk.
2. Trim, peel and grate the carrots. Roughly chop the peanuts. Combine the carrots, the milk mixture and the peanuts. Season the salad with salt and sprinkle with the snipped chives.

> **TIP**
> This carrot salad is perfectly suited as a cold lunchbox meal to take to work or school. Keep the salad in a well-sealed container and store in the fridge until ready to use.

NUTRITIONAL VALUES PER PORTION:
120 Cal • 4 g protein • 8 g fat • 8 g carbohydrate • 5 g dietary fibre • about 0.3 CE

Vegetable Salad with yoghurt

SERVES 2
250 g (8 oz) zucchini (courgettes)
1 large tomato
1 small onion
½ tsp finely chopped fresh ginger
150 g (5 oz) yoghurt (3.5% fat)
salt, pepper
1 tbsp chopped almonds
1 tbsp small parsley leaves
PREPARATION: about 15 mins

1. Wash the zucchini and the tomato, then chop into small pieces. Peel and halve the onion, then cut into thin strips.

2. Stir the ginger into the yoghurt. Combine with the zucchini and tomato pieces, onion strips and almonds. Season the salad with salt and pepper and stir in the parsley leaves.

TIP
Quick and easy to prepare, this is a perfect snack for anyone who likes (or needs) to eat several small meals throughout the day.

NUTRITIONAL VALUES PER PORTION:
100 Cal • 6 g protein • 6 g fat • 7 g carbohydrate • 2 g dietary fibre • about 0.3 CE

Orange Salad with onions

SERVES 2
2 small oranges
1 small white onion
1 red (Spanish) onion
2 spring onions
2 tbsp lemon juice
1½ tbsp olive oil
1 tsp finely chopped rosemary
salt, pepper
PREPARATION: about 20 mins
MARINATING: 1 hr

1. Peel the oranges and remove the flesh from between the membranes, catching the juice. Peel and halve the onions and cut into thin strips. Wash and trim the spring onions, then cut diagonally into thin rings.

2. Whisk the reserved orange juice, lemon juice, oil, chopped rosemary, salt and pepper to make a dressing. Combine the orange segments, onions and spring onions and cover evenly with the dressing. Cover and leave the salad to marinate for 1 hour. Check the seasoning again before serving.

SERVE WITH BREAD
Adjust the amount according to your daily carbohydrate requirements:
½ slice bread or ½ bread roll (about 25 g/¾ oz each) supply 0.7 CE.

TIP
This is an ideal lunchtime snack: the salad will stop any hunger pangs and keep the blood sugar level balanced.

NUTRITIONAL VALUES PER PORTION:
120 Cal • 1 g protein • 8 g fat • 12 g carbohydrate • 2 g dietary fibre • about 0.7 CE

Red Lentil Soup with parsley oil

SERVES 2

125 g (4 oz) red lentils
1 shallot
1 garlic clove
2½ tbsp olive oil
600 ml (20 fl oz/2½ cups) vegetable stock
1 bay leaf
4 sprigs parsley
1 pinch cayenne pepper
salt, pepper
1 tbsp lemon juice

PREPARATION: about 30 mins

1. Wash and drain the lentils. Peel and finely chop the shallot and the garlic.

2. In a saucepan, heat ½ tablespoon oil and fry the shallot and garlic until translucent. Add the lentils and briefly fry. Pour in the stock and add the bay leaf. Cover and simmer the lentil soup over low heat for about 20 minutes.

3. Wash and shake dry the parsley, then finely chop the leaves. Stir the cayenne pepper and the parsley into the remaining oil. Remove the bay leaf from the soup. Season the soup to taste with salt, pepper and lemon juice, then purée using a hand-held blender until smooth. Drizzle with the parsley oil and serve.

TIP

For a change, use fresh mint leaves instead of parsley when making the herb oil.

NUTRITIONAL VALUES PER PORTION:
375 Cal • 15 g protein • 16 g fat • 40 g carbohydrate • 10 g dietary fibre • about 2.7 CE

Barley & Vegetable Soup

SERVES 2

1 small onion
2 tsp rapeseed oil
50 g (1⅔ oz) pearl barley
1 clove
½ chopped parsley
600 ml (20 fl oz/2½ cups) vegetable stock
½ leek (about 100 g/3⅓ oz)
1 piece celeriac (about 60 g/2 oz)
salt, pepper
1 pinch freshly grated nutmeg
1 dash lemon juice
2 tsp sour cream
1 tbsp snipped chives

PREPARATION: about 45 mins

1. Peel and finely chop the onion. Heat the oil in a saucepan and fry the onion until translucent. Add the pearl barley and sauté briefly with the onion. Add the clove and parsley to season. Pour in the stock, cover and simmer the soup over low heat for about 25 minutes.

2. Meanwhile, trim the leek and halve lengthways. Wash thoroughly, then cut into thin rings. Peel and finely chop the celeriac. Add the vegetables to the barley, cover and continue simmering for about another 15 minutes.

3. If desired remove the garlic clove. Season the soup with salt, pepper, nutmeg and lemon juice. Add the sour cream and sprinkle with the chives.

VARIATION

You can make this soup with wholegrain barley: soak 50 g (1⅔ oz) barley grains overnight in 600 ml (20 fl oz/2½ cups) water, then cook in the soaking water for 1 hour. Add spices, stock and vegetables and finish cooking the soup.

NUTRITIONAL VALUES PER PORTION:
215 Cal • 4 g protein • 9 g fat • 26 g carbohydrate • 5 g dietary fibre • about 1.3 CE

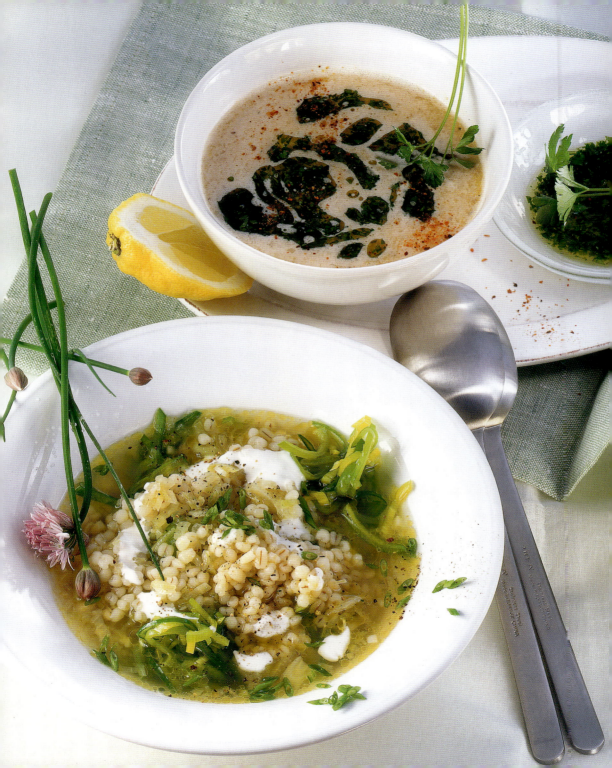

Jerusalem Artichoke Soup

SERVES 2

- 300 g (10 oz) Jerusalem artichokes (or 250 g/8 oz celeriac, see Tip)
- 2 spring onions
- 1 small garlic clove
- 1 small carrot
- 1 tbsp rapeseed oil
- 400 ml (14 fl oz/1¾ cups) vegetable stock
- 100 ml (3 fl oz/½ cup) low-fat milk (1.5% fat)
- herb-flavoured salt, pepper
- 1 dash lemon juice
- 2 tsp walnut oil (or olive oil)

PREPARATION: about 35 mins

1. Wash the Jerusalem artichokes. Cook, covered, for about 20 minutes in boiling water. Trim, wash and chop the spring onions. Peel and chop the garlic. Trim, peel and grate the carrot. Drain the artichokes, leave to cool a bit, then peel and dice.

2. Heat the oil in a saucepan. Fry the spring onions and garlic for 5 minutes. Add the artichokes and briefly fry. Pour in the stock and the milk and bring to the boil. Season with salt, pepper and lemon juice.

3. Finely purée the Jerusalem artichoke soup with a hand-held blender. Sprinkle with the carrot, drizzle with the walnut oil and serve piping hot.

TIP

Jerusalem artichokes are available in supermarket vegetable departments and organic stores. If you cannot find them, use celeriac instead. Peel the celeriac, cut into 1 cm (½ in) pieces and fry gently with the spring onions. Pour in the vegetable stock and the milk, cover and simmer for about 15 minutes, then season to taste.

NUTRITIONAL VALUES PER PORTION:
310 Cal • 14 g protein • 15 g fat • 28 g carbohydrate • 11 g dietary fibre • about 1.7 CE

French Onion Soup

SERVES 2

- 250 g (8 oz) brown onions
- 2 tbsp rapeseed oil
- 1 tbsp wholemeal flour
- 500 ml (16 fl oz/2 cups) chicken stock (or vegetable stock)
- 100 ml (3 fl oz/½ cup) dry white wine (or 100 ml/3 fl oz/½ cup vegetable stock plus 1 tsp lemon juice)
- salt, pepper
- 1 pinch ground caraway seeds
- 1 bay leaf
- 2 slices wholegrain toast
- 25 g (¾ oz) grated cheddar cheese
- 1 tsp chopped parsley

PREPARATION: about 30 mins

1. Peel, halve and finely slice the onions. Heat 1 tablespoon oil in a saucepan and fry the onions until lightly browned. Dust with flour and fry for a few minutes. Pour in the stock and the wine. Season with salt, pepper, caraway seeds and the bay leaf. Bring to the boil, cover and simmer for 15 minutes.

2. Preheat the oven to 225°C (435°F) or switch on the oven grill. Cut the bread slices into dice. Heat the remaining oil in a non-stick pan and fry the bread cubes in the pan until crispy all over. Combine the cheese and the parsley.

3. Transfer the soup to ovenproof soup bowls and put the bread cubes on top. Sprinkle with the cheese and parsley mixture. Bake in the oven (middle shelf, not suited for fan-forced ovens) or under a hot grill for about 3 minutes.

NUTRITIONAL VALUES PER PORTION:
345 Cal • 8 g protein • 18 g fat • 30 g carbohydrate • 6 g dietary fibre • 2 CE

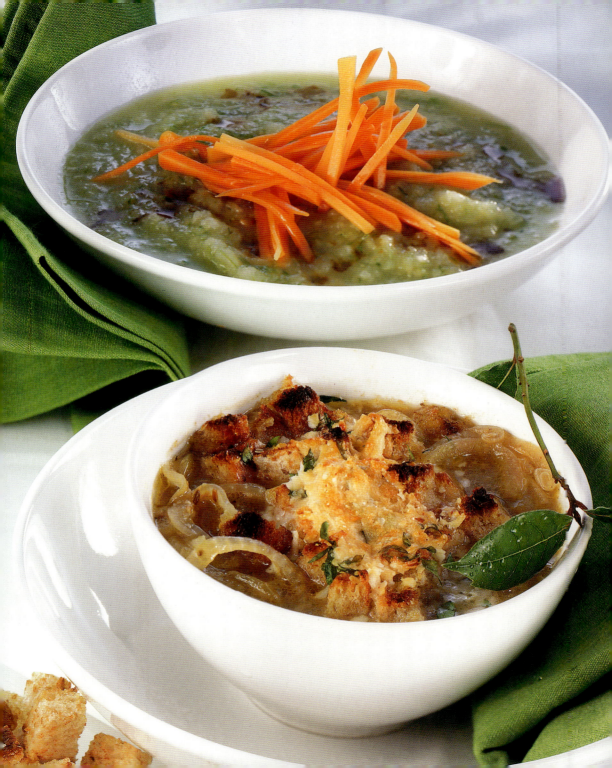

Asian Vegetable Soup

SERVES 2

50 g (1²⁄₃ oz) vermicelli
salt
1 garlic clove
2 tsp sunflower oil
500 ml (16 fl oz/2 cups) vegetable stock
200 g (6½ oz) frozen green beans
1 pack frozen or fresh soup vegetables (chopped onion, leek, celeriac, about 50 g/1²⁄₃ oz)
3 tbsp light soy sauce
1 tbsp lime juice (or lemon juice)
1 tsp sesame oil
pepper
1 tbsp fried onions (ready-made)
PREPARATION: about 25 mins

1. Cook the vermicelli as per packet instructions in plenty of salted water until al dente (firm to the bite). Drain and set aside.

2. Peel and finely chop the garlic. Heat the sunflower oil in a saucepan and gently fry the garlic until golden. Pour in the stock, and add the soup vegetables. Bring to the boil, cover and simmer over medium heat until the beans are cooked.

3. Season the soup with the soy sauce, lime juice, sesame oil and pepper.

4. Divide the vermicelli between two bowls. Pour in the hot vegetable soup. Sprinkle with the fried onions and serve.

TIP

You could also add lemon grass and coriander to this soup. Cook the lemon grass in the soup, and sprinkle the coriander leaves on top when ready to serve. Remove the lemon grass stalks before consuming.

NUTRITIONAL VALUES PER PORTION:
265 Cal • 8 g protein • 10 g fat • 34 g carbohydrate • 6 g dietary fibre • 2 CE

Quick Tomato Soup

SERVES 2

1 brown onion
1 garlic clove
1 small zucchini (courgette)
1 tbsp olive oil
200 g (6½ oz) tomato passata (tinned)
200 ml (7 fl oz/¾ cup) vegetable stock
salt, pepper
a few basil or parsley leaves
PREPARATION: about 20 mins

1. Peel and finely chop the onion and the garlic. Wash, trim and dice the zucchini.

2. Heat the oil in a saucepan, add the onion, garlic and zucchini and fry briefly. Add the tomatoes and the stock. Season with salt and pepper.

3. Bring to the boil, cover and simmer over low heat for about 7 minutes. Season the soup with salt and pepper. Sprinkle with a few basil leaves or some parsley and serve piping hot.

TIP

You can turn this soup into a light main course if you briefly heat 200 g (6½ oz) pre-cooked brown rice in the tomato soup. This will increase the overall CE value by about 1.3 units.

NUTRITIONAL VALUES PER PORTION:
105 Cal • 3 g protein • 6 g fat • 7 g carbohydrate • 2 g dietary fibre • 0 CE

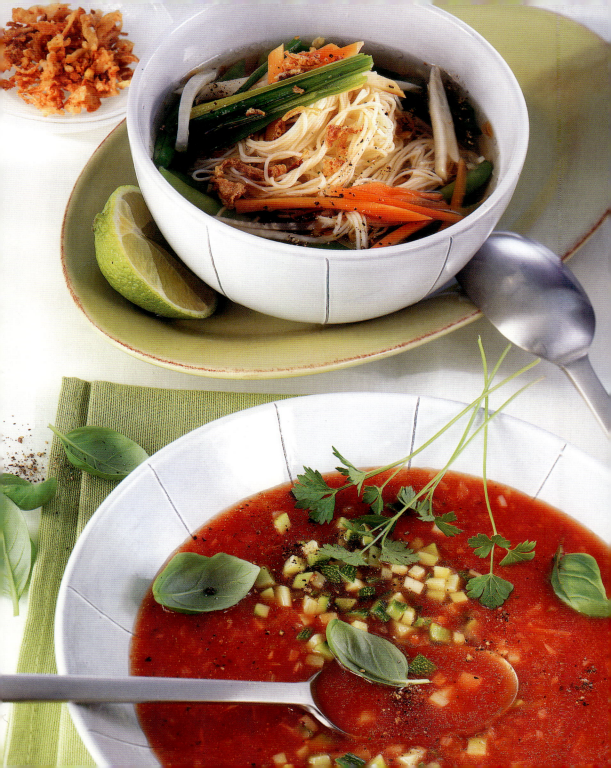

Warm Radicchio Salad

SERVES 2
350 g (11½ oz) radicchio
1 small red (Spanish) onion
1 orange
3 tbsp olive oil
2 tbsp balsamic vinegar
salt, pepper
30 g (1 oz) Parma ham
 (very thinly sliced)
20 g (⅔ oz) grated Parmesan
60 g (2 oz) wholemeal grissini
PREPARATION: about 20 mins

1. Trim, wash and shake dry the radicchio, then quarter lengthways, removing the core in a wedge shape. Peel and slice the onion. Peel the orange and cut the segments out from between the dividing membranes, while catching the juice.

2. Heat 2 tablespoons oil in a non-stick pan. Fry the radicchio quarters and the onion over medium heat for 5 minutes, turning occasionally. Add 1 tablespoon balsamic vinegar and the reserved orange juice and cook briefly.

3. Whisk the remaining balsamic vinegar with the rest of the oil. Season with salt and pepper. Arrange the radicchio, onion, orange fillets and Parma ham on the plates. Drizzle with the sauce and sprinkle with the Parmesan. Serve lukewarm with the grissini.

> **TIP**
> There are several varieties of radicchios. Some have small round heads, others have a more elongated shape. The best one to use for braising is the Treviso radicchio, which has a mildly bitter flavour and is good to use in this recipe.

NUTRITIONAL VALUES PER PORTION:
405 Cal • 14 g protein • 26 g fat • 33 g carbohydrate • 1 g dietary fibre • 2 CE

Broccoli with walnuts

SERVES 2
2 tbsp walnuts
 (or hazelnuts)
400 g (13 oz) broccoli
150 ml (5 fl oz/¾ cup)
 vegetable stock
1 small onion
1 tbsp lemon juice
½ tbsp walnut oil
 (or olive oil)
salt, pepper
PREPARATION: about 20 mins

1. Roughly chop the walnuts and dry-roast in a non-stick pan without fat until golden. Take out and set aside. Trim the broccoli, separate into small florets and rinse with water. Peel the broccoli stems and slice thinly.

2. Bring the stock to the boil in a frying pan. Add the broccoli florets and stem slices and cook for 5 minutes until firm to the bite. Peel and finely chop the onion. Stir together 3–4 tablespoons broccoli stock with the lemon juice, oil and the onion to make a sauce. Season generously with salt and pepper. Drain the broccoli and leave to cool a little.

3. Arrange the warm broccoli on serving plates. Drizzle with the sauce and sprinkle the nuts on top. Serve the vegetable dish lukewarm or cold.

> **SERVE WITH BREAD**
> Adjust the amount according to your daily carbohydrate requirements: ½ slice bread or ½ bread roll (about 25 g/¾ oz each) supply 0.7 CE.

NUTRITIONAL VALUES PER PORTION:
140 Cal • 6 g protein • 10 g fat • 7 g carbohydrate • 5 g dietary fibre • 0 CE

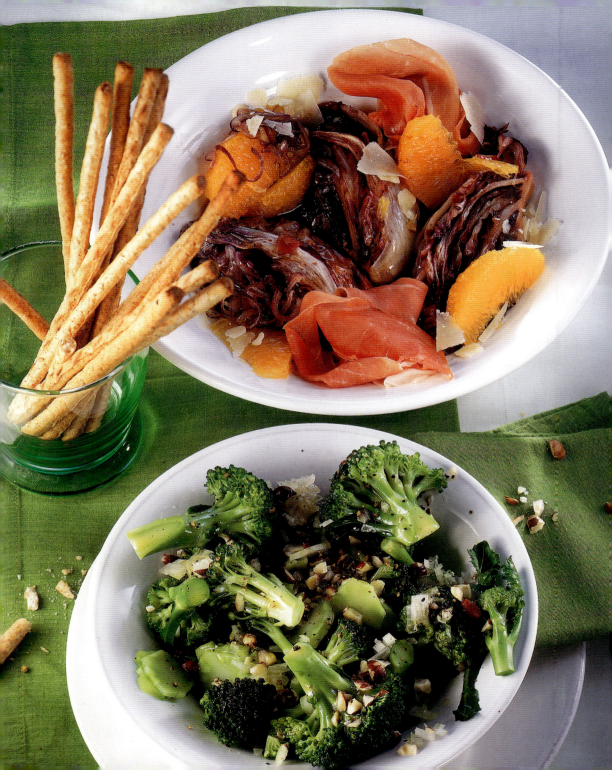

Mediterranean Vegetables

SERVES 2

400 g (13 oz) mixed vegetables (e.g. celery, capsicum, zucchini and fennel bulb)

1 sprig rosemary

1 sprig thyme

½ bunch flat-leaf parsley

½ organic lemon

1 tbsp olive oil

4 tbsp vegetable stock

salt, pepper

PREPARATION: about 25 mins

1. Wash and trim the vegetables, then cut into large chunks. Wash and shake dry the rosemary, thyme and parsley. Reserve some of the herbs and finely chop the rest. Brush the lemon under hot water, then cut into thin wedges.

2. Combine the vegetables with the herbs, lemon wedges, oil and stock. Heat a large (griddle) pan and braise the vegetables in the liquid for about 10 minutes until firm to the bite, turning occasionally.

3. Remove the lemon wedges and season the vegetables with salt and pepper. Garnish with the reserved herbs.

> **TIP**
>
> You can serve this vegetable dish on its own as a light snack, or as a side dish with grilled meat or fish. Jacket potatoes would be a tasty addition. An unpeeled potato weighing 200 g (6½ oz) baked in the oven wrapped in foil will provide about 2.3 CE.

NUTRITIONAL VALUES PER PORTION:

90 Cal • 3 g protein • 6 g fat • 5 g carbohydrate • 6 g dietary fibre • 0 CE

Cauliflower with a curried yoghurt sauce

SERVES 2

500 g (1 lb) cauliflower

salt

2 tbsp lemon juice

150 g (5 oz) low-fat yoghurt (1.5% fat)

1 tsp vegetable oil

2 tbsp chopped parsley

1 tsp mild curry powder

pepper

PREPARATION: about 20 mins

1. Trim the cauliflower, separate into florets and rinse with water. Cook in plenty of salted water with 1 tablespoon lemon juice for 5–7 minutes until firm to the bite. Drain, rinse under cold water and drain again.

2. Whisk together the yoghurt, oil and remaining lemon juice. Stir in the parsley. Season to taste with ½–1 teaspoon curry powder, salt and pepper.

3. Serve the cauliflower lukewarm or cold in the sauce. Otherwise leave the cauliflower to draw flavour in the sauce for 10 minutes.

> **SERVE WITH BREAD**
>
> Adjust the amount according to your daily carbohydrate requirements: ½ slice bread or ½ bread roll (about 25 g/¾ oz each) supply 0.7 CE.
>
> **VARIATION**
>
> Cauliflower can also be consumed raw. Trim and wash, then coarsely grate the cauliflower. Combine immediately with the curry sauce. This salad goes well alongside grilled poultry or fish dishes.

NUTRITIONAL VALUES PER PORTION:

95 Cal • 6 g protein • 4 g fat • 7 g carbohydrate • 5 g dietary fibre • 0 CE

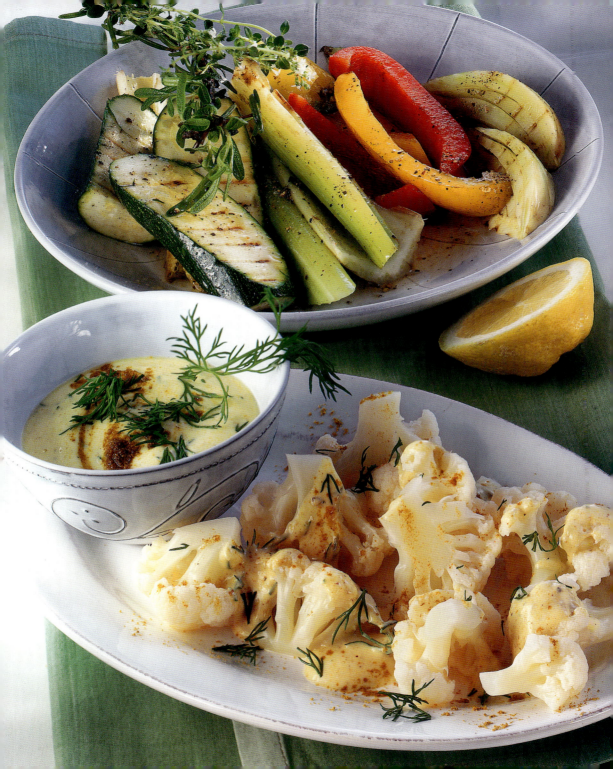

Fennel & Tomatoes with Parmesan

SERVES 2

2 fennel bulbs (about 400 g/13 oz)
200 g (6½ oz) tomatoes
2 tsp olive oil
2 tbsp vegetable stock
salt
coarsely ground pepper
40 g (1½ oz) chunk of Parmesan

PREPARATION: about 25 mins

1. Wash and trim the fennel. Reserve the tender green parts. Quarter the bulbs lengthways, then grate into thin slices.

2. Wash and slice the tomatoes. Roughly chop the fennel greens. Whisk the oil and the stock with a little salt and pepper to make a salad dressing.

3. Arrange the tomato and fennel slices on two serving plates and drizzle with the dressing. Sprinkle with the fennel greens and grate the Parmesan over the top of the salad.

TIP

This Italian-style vegetarian side salad ensures that your blood sugar levels will stay balanced in between meals.

NUTRITIONAL VALUES PER PORTION:
175 Cal • 12 g protein • 11 g fat • 6 g carbohydrate • 8 g dietary fibre • 0 CE

Spinach in a sesame sauce

SERVES 2

250 g (7½ oz) frozen spinach
2 tsp hulled sesame seeds
2 tbsp tahini (sesame paste, ready-made)
2 tbsp light soy sauce
½ tsp sugar
salt

PREPARATION: about 20 mins

1. Prepare spinach as per packet instructions. Briefly dry-roast the sesame seeds in a non-stick pan without fat.

2. Whisk together the tahini with the soy sauce, sugar and 2–4 tablespoons water until you have a smooth paste. Drain the spinach, squeezing out any excess liquid. Stir the sesame sauce into the spinach. Season with salt and sprinkle with the roasted sesame seeds.

TIP

This Asian-inspired dish tastes good as a snack or if served as a starter, for example with the Duck Breast with Broccoli and Nuts recipe on page 98.

NUTRITIONAL VALUES PER PORTION:
155 Cal • 7 g protein • 10 g fat • 10 g carbohydrate • 1 g dietary fibre • about 0.3 CE

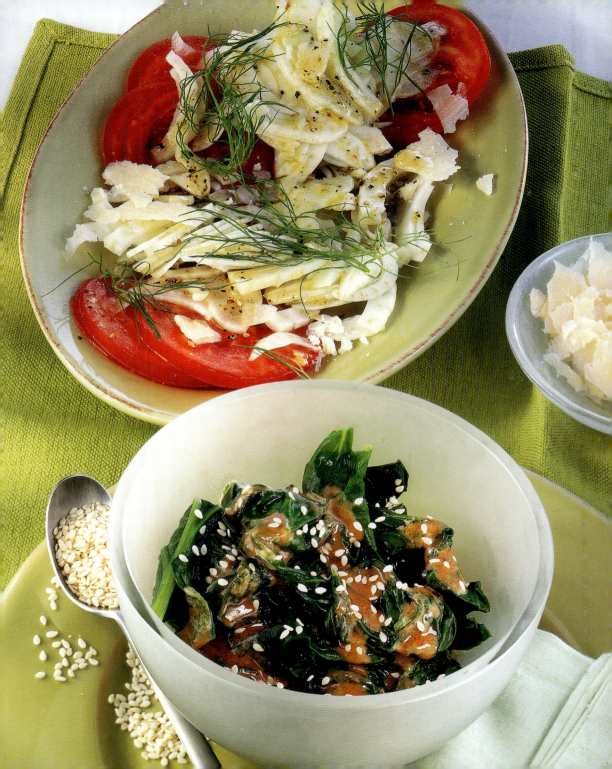

Eggplant bake

SERVES 2

1 eggplant (aubergine, about 300 g/10 oz)
2 tbsp olive oil
300 g (10 oz) tomatoes
1 garlic clove
30 g (1 oz) grated Pecorino
1 tbsp chopped basil
2 slices wholemeal bread with sunflower seeds (60 g/2 oz each)
salt, pepper
50 ml (2 fl oz/¼ cup) vegetable stock

PREPARATION: about 25 mins
BAKING: about 35 mins

1. Trim and wash the eggplant, then cut crossways into ½ cm (¼ in slices). In a non-stick pan, heat 1 tablespoon oil and fry the eggplant slices, a few at a time, on both sides.

2. Wash and slice the tomatoes. Peel and finely slice the garlic. Combine the garlic, cheese and basil. Preheat the oven to 200°C (390°F) /180°C (355°F) fan-forced (middle shelf). Meanwhile, brush an ovenproof dish with a little oil.

3. Cut the bread into squares of about 3 cm (1¼ in). Layer the eggplant and tomato slices as well as the bread in the baking dish (see picture). Season with salt and pepper, then sprinkle the cheese and herb mixture over the top. Drizzle with the stock and the remaining oil. Bake in the oven for about 35 minutes. Garnish with basil and serve.

NUTRITIONAL VALUES PER PORTION:
410 Cal • 13 g protein • 26 g fat • 29 g carbohydrate • 7 g dietary fibre • 2 CE

Kohlrabi & Potato Bake

SERVES 2

600 g (1 lb 3 oz) kohlrabi (or turnip)
200 g (6½ oz) waxy potatoes
1 tbsp chopped parsley
salt, pepper
½ tsp oil
100 ml (3 fl oz/½ cup) soy cream
250 ml (8 fl oz/1 cup) low-fat milk (1.5% fat)
1 pinch freshly grated nutmeg

PREPARATION: about 25 mins
BAKING: about 35 mins

1. Peel and trim the kohlrabi and the potatoes. Reserve the tender kohlrabi greens. Quarter the kohlrabi. Cut the kohlrabi quarters and the potatoes into thin slices (use a vegetable slicer if you have one). Combine the kohlrabi, potatoes and parsley, and season with salt and pepper.

2. Preheat the oven to 200°C (390°F) /180°C (355°F) fan-forced (middle shelf). Brush a shallow ovenproof dish with oil. Place the kohlrabi and potato mixture in the dish and smooth over the top. Stir the soy cream with the milk and season generously with salt, pepper and nutmeg. Pour evenly over the vegetables.

3. Bake in the oven for about 35 minutes until golden. Sprinkle with chopped kohlrabi greens and serve.

TIP
Soy cream is a plant-based alternative to crème fraîche or cream. Soy cream is also free from cholesterol as well as being rich in healthy polyunsaturated fatty acids.

NUTRITIONAL VALUES PER PORTION:
280 Cal • 11 g protein • 12 g fat • 32 g carbohydrate • 6 g dietary fibre • 2 CE

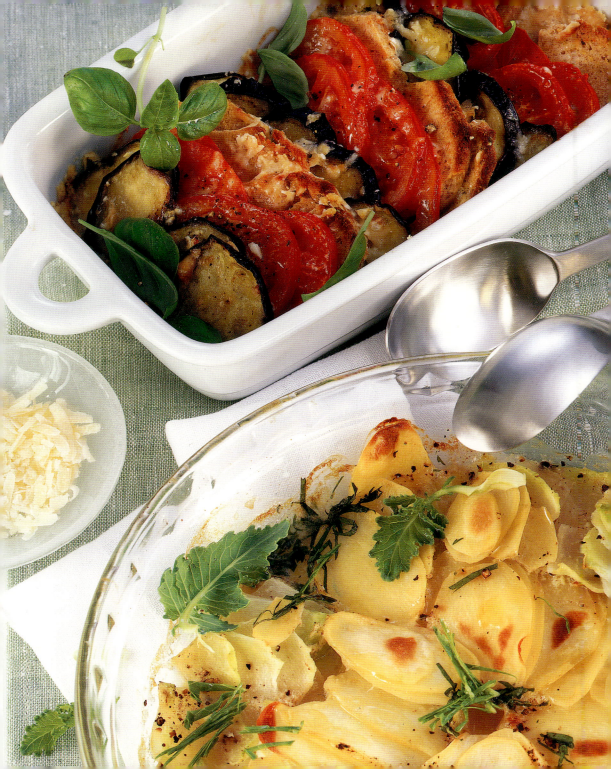

Cheesy Zucchini Parcels

SERVES 2

150 g (5 oz) feta cheese

2 zucchini (courgettes)

salt

2 tsp olive oil

pepper

1 pinch sweet paprika

200 g (6½ oz) chopped tomatoes with herbs (tinned)

PREPARATION: about 30 mins

1. Preheat the oven to 175°C (345°F) /160°C (320°F) fan-forced (middle shelf). Cut the cheese into four long strips of the same size. Wash and trim the zucchini, then cut lengthways into thin slices. Blanch the slices in boiling salted water for 20 seconds, rinse under cold water and drain.

2. Wrap 2–3 zucchini slices around the cheese strips. Place the parcels in an ovenproof dish. Season the oil with salt, pepper and sweet paprika and brush the parcels evenly with the mixture. Bake in the oven for about 15 minutes.

3. Meanwhile heat the tomatoes. Cut the remaining zucchini slices into strips and add to the tomatoes. Season the sauce with salt and pepper. Arrange the cheese and zucchini parcels on top of the tomato sauce and serve.

> **SERVE WITH BREAD**
> Adjust the amount according to your daily carbohydrate requirements: ½ slice bread or ½ bread roll (about 25 g/¾ oz each) supply 0.7 CE.

NUTRITIONAL VALUES PER PORTION:
260 Cal • 24 g protein • 18 g fat • 6 g carbohydrate • 1 g dietary fibre • 0 CE

Savoury Baked Apples

SERVES 2

150 g (5 oz) brown onions

1 sprig sage

2 red apples (200 g/6½ oz each)

1 tsp lemon juice

2 tsp reduced-fat butter

pepper

PREPARATION: about 20 mins
BAKING: 25 MINS

> **TIP**
> These apples could also be served as a side dish with pan-fried meat.

1. Preheat the oven to 175°C/160°C fan-forced (middle shelf). Peel and finely dice the onions. Wash and shake dry the sage and chop the leaves into strips.

2. Wash and pat dry the apples, then cut off a top on each stem side. Using an apple corer, remove the core, without completely cutting through the apples. Make the opening slightly larger and brush with lemon juice. Finely chop the apple flesh that has been removed.

3. Melt 1 teaspoon reduced-fat butter in a non-stick frying pan. Gently sauté the onions and sage until the onions are lightly browned. Stir in the chopped apple. Season the onion and apple mixture with pepper and place inside the hollowed out apples. Cover the apples with the apple tops.

4. Line the base of a small ovenproof dish with foil. Place the apples in the dish and brush with the remaining butter. Bake in the oven for about 25 minutes.

NUTRITIONAL VALUES PER PORTION:
140 Cal • 1 g protein • 3 g fat • 29 g carbohydrate • 6 g dietary fibre • 2 CE

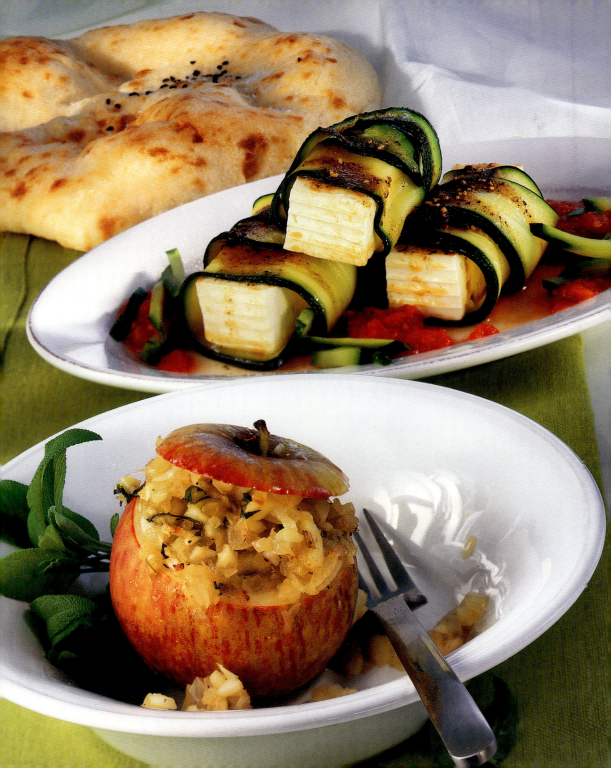

Vegetable Rice with hard-boiled eggs

SERVES 2

100 g (3⅓ oz) brown long-grain rice (parboiled)
150 g (5 oz) frozen spinach
150 g (5 oz) leeks
2 carrots
1 kohlrabi (or turnip)
1 small onion
1 tbsp rapeseed oil
salt, pepper
100 ml (3 fl oz/½ cup) vegetable stock
2 eggs
2 tbsp yoghurt (3.5% fat)
1 tbsp chopped parsley

PREPARATION: about 35 mins

1. Cook the rice and the spinach as per individual packet instructions. Leave both to drain.

2. Trim the leeks and slice lengthways; thoroughly wash them and diagonally cut into thin slices. Trim and peel the carrots and the kohlrabi. Cut the carrots into diagonal slices and the kohlrabi into sticks. Peel and finely chop the onion.

3. Heat the oil in a saucepan. Sauté the onion, leek, carrots and kohlrabi for 5 minutes. Season with salt and pepper. Pour in the stock, cover and cook the vegetables for a further 5–7 minutes.

4. Meanwhile cook the eggs for 7 minutes until they are just hard. Stir the spinach and the yoghurt into the vegetables. Gently combine the rice, vegetables and parsley. Season with salt and pepper and arrange on serving plates. Rinse the eggs under cold water, shell and halve them and place on top of the rice.

TIP
Medium-sized eggs are perfect when only just hard, with a waxy soft centre, after 7 minutes. For small or large eggs you'll need to increase or decrease the cooking time by about 1 minute.

NUTRITIONAL VALUES PER PORTION:
370 Cal • 15 g protein • 11 g fat • 50 g carbohydrate • 6 g dietary fibre • about 3.3 CE

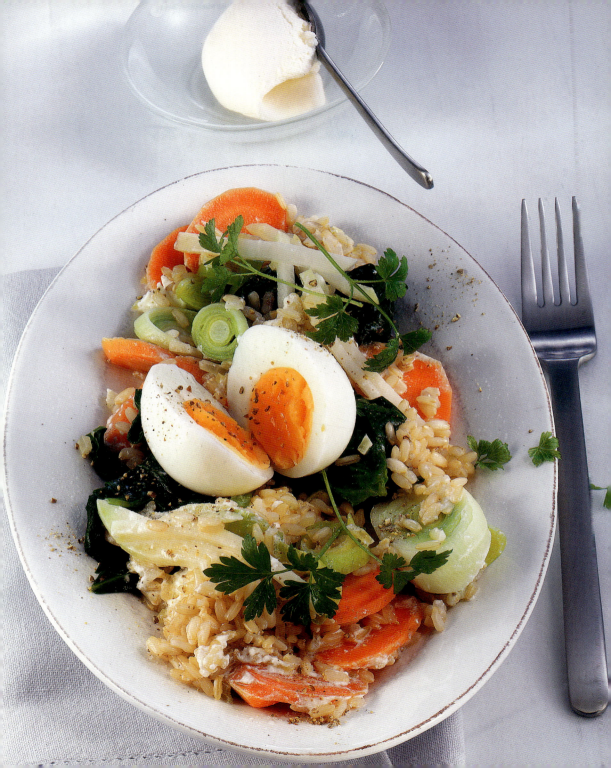

Spinach Dumplings with tomato sauce

SERVES 2

250 g (8 oz) frozen spinach
5 slices wholegrain toast
2 shallots
1 garlic clove
2 tbsp olive oil
1 egg
5 tbsp low-fat milk (1.5% fat)
30 g (1 oz) wholegrain breadcrumbs
salt, pepper
1 pinch freshly grated nutmeg
½ tsp dried oregano
1 tin chopped tomatoes (400 g/13 oz)

PREPARATION: about 40 mins

1. Defrost the spinach. Cut the bread into 1 cm (½ in) pieces. Peel and finely chop 1 shallot and the garlic. Heat 1 tablespoon oil in a frying pan and fry the shallot and garlic until translucent. Add the bread pieces and fry for 5 minutes. Remove and leave to cool.

2. Stir the egg into the milk, pour over the bread mixture and leave to soak for 5 minutes. Squeeze out the spinach and finely chop it. Add the spinach and the breadcrumbs to the bread pieces. Season with salt, pepper and nutmeg. Knead everything into a dough and shape into 8 dumplings. In a saucepan, bring salted water to the boil. Add the dumplings, cover and simmer over low heat for about 10 minutes.

3. Peel and finely slice the other shallot. Heat the remaining oil and fry the shallot until translucent. Add the oregano and the tomatoes and simmer for 5 minutes. Season with salt and pepper. Remove then drain the dumplings. Arrange in the tomato sauce and serve.

NUTRITIONAL VALUES PER PORTION:
415 Cal • 19 g protein • 16 g fat • 47 g carbohydrate • 5 g dietary fibre • about 3.3 CE

Millet with ratatouille

SERVES 2

1 red capsicum (pepper)
2 small zucchini (courgettes)
1 small eggplant (aubergine)
1 onion
300 ml (10 fl oz/1¼ cups) vegetable stock
120 g (4 oz) millet
2 tbsp olive oil
250 g (8 oz) tomatoes
1 garlic clove
2 tsp chopped thyme
1 tsp chopped rosemary
salt, black pepper
2 tbsp dry rosé wine (or vegetable stock)
a few basil leaves

PREPARATION: about 45 mins

1. Quarter and trim the capsicum, then cut crossways into strips. Wash and trim the zucchini and the eggplant, then cut into 1 cm (½ in) dice. Peel and chop the onion. Bring the stock to the boil and cook the millet for about 25 minutes.

2. Meanwhile, heat 1 tablespoon oil in a saucepan. Fry the eggplant for 10 minutes, turning a few times. Heat the remaining oil in a non-stick pan and briefly fry the onion. Add the zucchini and the capsicum and fry for 5 minutes, turning a few times.

3. Wash and roughly dice the tomatoes. Peel and finely chop the garlic. Season the eggplant with thyme, rosemary and garlic. Stir in the tomatoes and the zucchini and capsicum mixture. Season the ratatouille with salt and pepper, and pour in the wine. Cover and braise the vegetables for about 10 minutes. Arrange the millet on a plate with the vegetables, garnish with a few basil leaves and serve.

NUTRITIONAL VALUES PER PORTION:
410 Cal • 10 g protein • 15 g fat • 55 g carbohydrate • 11 g dietary fibre • about 3.3 CE

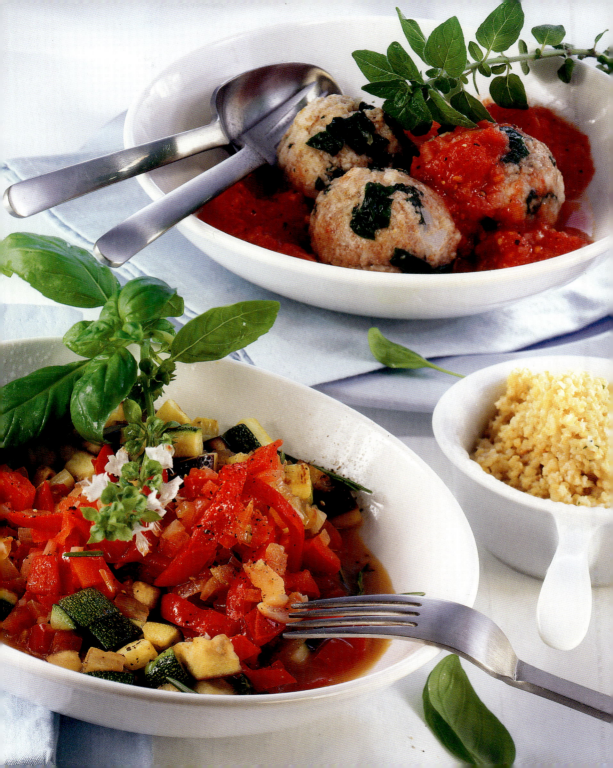

Cabbage Rolls with bulgur filling

SERVES 2

1 shallot
1 garlic clove
2 tbsp olive oil
100 g (3⅓ oz) bulgur
1 tbsp tomato paste
¼ tsp sweet paprika
½ tsp chopped oregano
salt, pepper
300 ml (10 fl oz/1¼ cups) vegetable stock
8 pointed cabbage leaves
20 g (⅔ oz) grated Parmesan
2 tbsp chopped flat-leaf parsley
2 tsp lemon juice
75 ml (2½ fl oz/⅓ cup) freshly squeezed orange juice
1 tbsp sour cream
1 tsp wholemeal flour
1 pinch saffron powder
a few pink peppercorns

PREPARATION: about 50 mins

1. Peel and finely chop the shallot and garlic. In a saucepan heat ½ tablespoon oil and fry shallot and garlic until translucent. Add the bulgur and tomato paste. Season with sweet paprika, oregano, salt and pepper. Pour in 200 ml (7 fl oz/ ¾ cup) stock, cover and cook the bulgur for about 15 minutes.

2. Wash the cabbage leaves. Bring plenty of lightly salted water to the boil and blanch the leaves for about 1 minute, then drain and rinse under cold water. Cut out the hard central stems in a wedge shape.

3. Stir the Parmesan, 1 tablespoon parsley and 1 teaspoon lemon juice into the bulgur. Spread out the cabbage leaves on a work surface. Place the filling into the middle of each leaf. Fold the leaves around the filling and make each leaf into a roll. Tie with kitchen string.

4. Heat the remaining oil in a saucepan. Fry the cabbage rolls in the oil. Pour in the remaining stock, cover and braise the rolls over low heat for about 25 minutes.

5. Whisk together the orange juice, sour cream and flour. Lift out the cabbage rolls. Pour the juice mixture into the frying juices, heat stirring constantly and simmer for about 3 minutes. Season the sauce with saffron, salt, pepper and the remaining lemon juice. Stir in the rest of the parsley and briefly reheat the cabbage rolls in the sauce. Sprinkle with pink peppercorns and serve immediately.

TIP
The season for pointed cabbage is fairly short, but you can fill the leaves of white or Savoy cabbage or silverbeet with the bulgur instead.

NUTRITIONAL VALUES PER PORTION:
395 Cal • 12 g protein • 17 g fat • 50 g carbohydrate • 16 g dietary fibre • about 3.3 CE

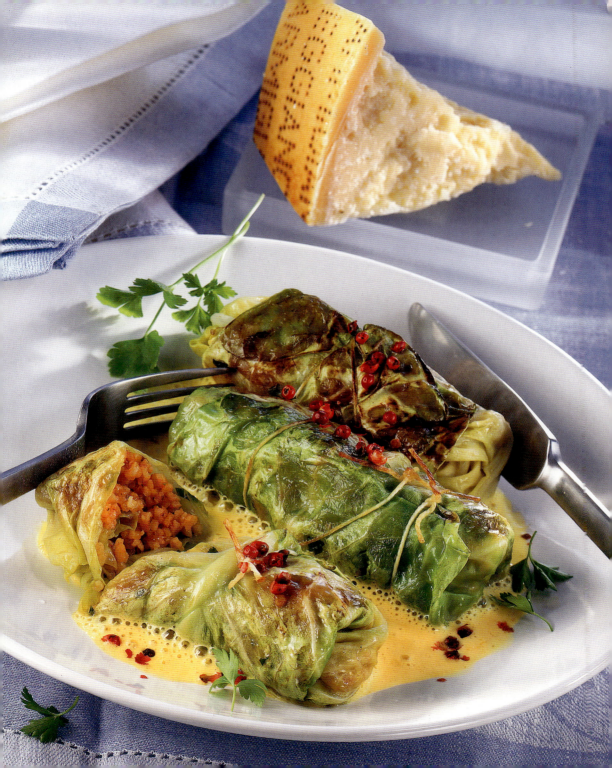

Spaghetti with pumpkin seed & herb pesto

SERVES 2

1 bunch flat-leaf parsley
2 garlic cloves
2 tbsp pumpkin seeds
40 g (1½ oz) grated Parmesan
2 tbsp pumpkin seed oil
2 tbsp rapeseed oil
salt, black pepper
160 g (5⅓ oz) spaghetti

PREPARATION: about 25 mins

1. Wash and shake dry the parsley, then finely chop the leaves. Peel and finely chop the garlic. Briefly dry-roast the pumpkin seeds in a non-stick frying pan without fat.

2. Reserve 2 teaspoons Parmesan. Using a hand-held blender chop the remaining Parmesan, parsley, garlic and pumpkin seeds.

3. Add both oils, a little at a time, in a thin stream. Season the pesto with salt and pepper to taste. Cook the spaghetti in plenty of salted water as per the packet instructions until firm to the bite. Drain, stirring 2 tablespoons of the cooking water into the pesto. Serve the spaghetti with the pesto and sprinkle the Parmesan on top.

VARIATION

Try a different pesto: 1 bunch parsley, 2 garlic cloves, 40 g (1½ oz) grated Parmesan, 2 tbsp ground almonds and 4 tbsp rapeseed oil.

NUTRITIONAL VALUES PER PORTION:
605 Cal • 22 g protein • 30 g fat • 63 g carbohydrate • 2 g dietary fibre • 4 CE

Spinach-filled Cannelloni

SERVES 2

225 g (7½ oz) frozen spinach
100 g (3⅓ oz) zucchini (courgette)
125 g (4 oz) low-fat cream cheese
1 small egg
1 tsp dried thyme
1 garlic clove
salt, pepper
1 pinch freshly grated nutmeg
1 tsp oil
12 wholemeal cannelloni (120 g/4 oz, precooked)
1 onion
370 g (12 oz) chopped tomatoes with herbs (tinned)
100 ml (3 fl oz/½ cup) vegetable stock
2 tbsp grated Parmesan

PREPARATION: about 35 mins
BAKING: about 35 mins

1. Cook the spinach as per the packet instructions. Drain, roughly chop and leave to cool, then squeeze out any moisture. Wash, trim and finely chop the zucchini. Place the spinach, zucchini, cream cheese, egg and thyme in a bowl. Peel then crush the garlic and add to the mixture. Stir to combine and season with salt, pepper and nutmeg.

2. Preheat the oven to 200°C (390°F) /180°C (355°F) fan-forced (middle shelf). Brush an ovenproof dish with oil. Using a teaspoon, fill the spinach mixture into the cannelloni. Place the cannelloni into the dish.

3. Peel and finely chop the onion. Stir together the tomatoes, stock and onion. Season the sauce with salt and pepper and spread on top of the cannelloni. Bake for about 35 minutes in the oven until the cannelloni are soft and lightly browned. Check if they are cooked using the tip of a knife. Sprinkle with the Parmesan.

TIP

After removing from the oven, leave the cannelloni for 5-10 minutes to rest before serving so the soft filling can firm up slightly.

NUTRITIONAL VALUES PER PORTION:
425 Cal • 30 g protein • 11 g fat • 51 g carbohydrate • 6 g dietary fibre • about 3.3 CE

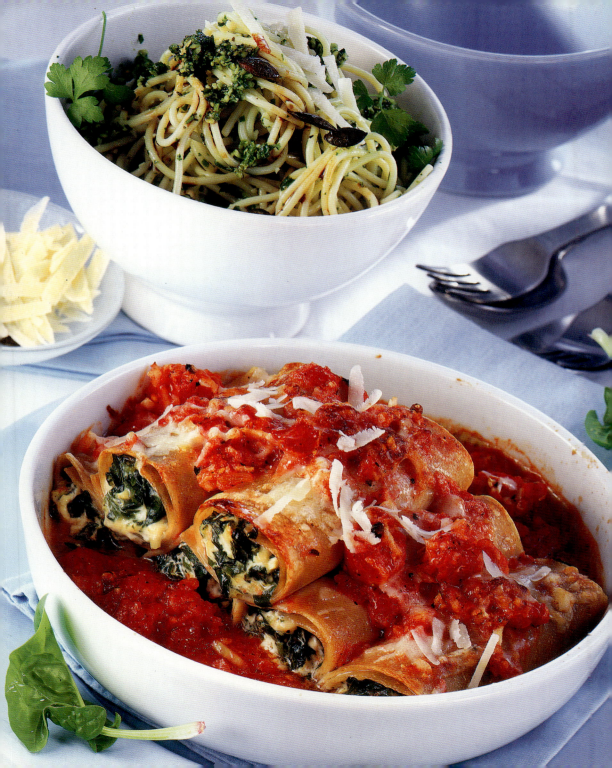

Pizza with artichokes

SERVES 2
FOR THE DOUGH
10 g (½ oz) fresh yeast
150 g (5 oz) wholemeal flour
salt
1½ tbsp olive oil

FOR THE TOPPING
500 g (1 lb) tomatoes
4 preserved artichoke hearts
50 g (1²/₃ oz) blue cheese
   (e.g. gorgonzola)
6 black pitted olives
salt, pepper
1 tbsp olive oil
2 tbsp vegetable stock
1 tbsp grated Parmesan
a few basil leaves

PREPARATION: about 30 mins
BAKING: about 20 mins

1. To make the dough, dissolve the yeast in 90 ml (2¾ fl oz/⅓ cup) lukewarm water. Stir in the flour, ¼ teaspoon salt and 1 tablespoon oil until smooth. Knead the mixture until you have a smooth and elastic dough. Brush a round tart or pizza dish (about 22 cm/8½ in diameter) with the remaining oil. Roll out the dough on the work surface; press into the dish.

2. Preheat the oven to 220°C (430°F) /200°C (390°F) fan-forced (bottom shelf). Briefly dip the tomatoes into boiling water, then remove the skins and cut in half and deseed. Drain the artichokes and chop into small slices. Slice the cheese and halve the olives.

3. Arrange the tomatoes, artichokes and cheese on the dough base. Season with salt and pepper. Stir the oil into the stock and drizzle over.

4. Bake the pizza in the oven for about 20 minutes. Sprinkle with the Parmesan and some basil leaves. This goes well with a green salad with a yoghurt dressing.

VARIATION
If you like, you can replace the artichokes with 150 g (5 oz) small broccoli florets, blanched in hot water.

NUTRITIONAL VALUES PER PORTION:
500 Cal • 19 g protein • 25 g fat • 50 g carbohydrate • 15 g dietary fibre • about 3.3 CE

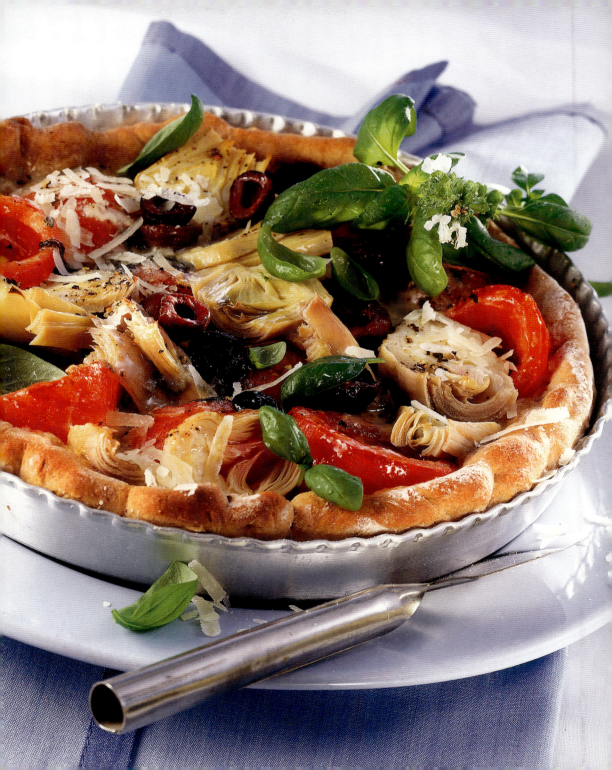

Wok Vegetables with glass noodles

SERVES 2

50 g (1²⁄₃ oz) Chinese glass noodles
1 small Chinese cabbage (about 300 g/10 oz)
1 red capsicum (pepper)
1 large onion
1 garlic clove
1 tbsp vegetable oil
1 tbsp sesame oil
salt, pepper
3 tbsp light soy sauce
cayenne pepper
50 ml (2 fl oz/¼ cup) vegetable stock
2 tbsp roasted unsalted peanuts

PREPARATION: about 30 mins

1. Place the glass noodles into a bowl, cover with warm water and leave for 10 minutes to expand. Drain and cut into short lengths, using scissors.

2. Meanwhile, wash and trim the Chinese cabbage, then cut into 2,5 cm (1 in) wide strips. Wash and trim the capsicum and cut into strips. Peel the onion and the garlic. Cut the onion into eighths, separating the layers, and finely chop the garlic.

3. Heat both the oils in a wok or a large frying pan. Add the onion and capsicum and fry for 3 minutes, stirring constantly. Stir in the garlic and the cabbage and fry for another 4 minutes. Season with salt and pepper.

4. Stir the soy sauce, salt and a little cayenne pepper into the stock. Stir the glass noodles into the vegetables and pour in the stock. Briefly bring to the boil, stirring constantly. Check the seasoning. Roughly chop the peanuts and sprinkle over the top. Serve hot.

NUTRITIONAL VALUES PER PORTION:
250 Cal • 11 g protein • 11 g fat • 29 g carbohydrate • 7 g dietary fibre • about 1.7 CE

Fried Vegetables with parsley sauce

SERVES 2

300 g (10 oz) small new potatoes
800 g (1lb 10oz) mixed vegetables (e.g. brussels sprouts, broccoli, carrots and savoy cabbage)
salt
100 g (3⅓ oz) button mushrooms
1 tbsp olive oil
4 cherry tomatoes
1 tbsp parsley leaves
1 tbsp chopped parsley
pepper
1 large egg
150 ml (5 fl oz/¾ cup) vegetable stock
1-2 tbsp white balsamic vinegar

PREPARATION: about 40 mins

1. Cook the unpeeled potatoes in water for 15–20 minutes. Meanwhile, wash the vegetables and trim or peel them, then cut into bite-sized pieces. Cook each vegetable separately in boiling salted water until firm to the bite. Drain, rinse in cold water and leave to drain again.

2. Brush and halve the mushrooms. Heat the oil in a non-stick pan. Fry all the vegetables and the mushrooms, a few at a time, in the oil until golden. Wash and halve the tomatoes. Stir into the vegetables together with the parsley leaves and season with salt and pepper. Slip the skins off the potatoes. Cover potatoes and vegetables and keep warm.

3. In a metal bowl, stir together the egg, 100 ml (3 fl oz/½ cup) stock, the balsamic vinegar and a little salt and pepper. Beat everything into a creamy sauce over a lightly boiling bain marie. Fold in the chopped parsley and check the seasoning.

4. Arrange the vegetables on plates and drizzle with the remaining stock. Serve with the parsley sauce and the potatoes.

NUTRITIONAL VALUES PER PORTION:
325 Cal • 19 g protein • 10 g fat • 37 g carbohydrate • 18 g dietary fibre • about 2.3 CE

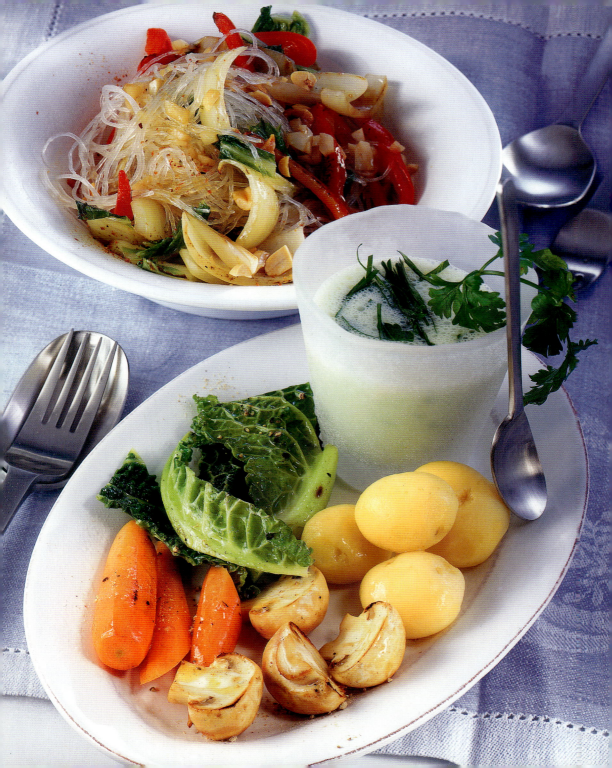

MAIN COURSES - VEGETARIAN

Turnip Quiche

SERVES 2
FOR THE QUICHE
2 floury potatoes
1 tsp oil
100 g (3⅓ oz) wholemeal flour
1 level tsp baking powder
10 g (½ oz) reduced-fat butter
salt
2 tbsp milk (1.5% fat)
FOR THE TOPPING
300 g (10 oz) turnip
pepper
30 g (1 oz) gorgonzola
100 g (3⅓ oz) low-fat
   yoghurt (1.5% fat)
1 small egg
1 tbsp parsley leaves
PREPARATION: about 45 mins
BAKING: about 30 mins

1. To make the quiche, wash the potatoes and cook (unpeeled) in water for about 25 minutes. Drain, leave to cool briefly, then peel off the skins. Weigh 100 g (3 oz) potatoes and push them through a potato ricer while still hot. Preheat the oven to 180°C (355°F) /160°C (320°F) fan-forced (bottom shef). Brush a loose-bottom tin (18 cm/7 in diameter) with the oil.

2. Combine the flour and the baking powder. Quickly knead the pressed potatoes with the flour, the butter, 1 pinch salt and the milk to make a dough. Roll out the dough on a lightly floured work surface or between two sheets of cling film to ½ cm (¼ in) thick. Line the base of the tin, forming an edge about 3 cm (1¼ in) high. Frick the base several times with a fork (do not press all the way through).

3. To make the topping, trim, peel and quarter the turnip and cut into very thin slices. Lightly season with salt and pepper. Wash 3–4 tender turnip leaves and finely chop them. Mash the cheese with a fork, then combine with the yoghurt, egg and chopped turnip leaves. Season with pepper.

4. Stir the turnip into the yoghurt mixture and spread this on top of the dough base. Bake in the oven for about 30 minutes. Leave the quiche to rest briefly before serving, then cut into slices. Sprinkle with parsley leaves and serve. A mixed leaf salad with a herb vinaigrette would make a tasty accompaniment.

NUTRITIONAL VALUES PER PORTION:
435 Cal • 20 g protein • 12 g fat • 62 g carbohydrate • 7 g dietary fibre • 4 CE

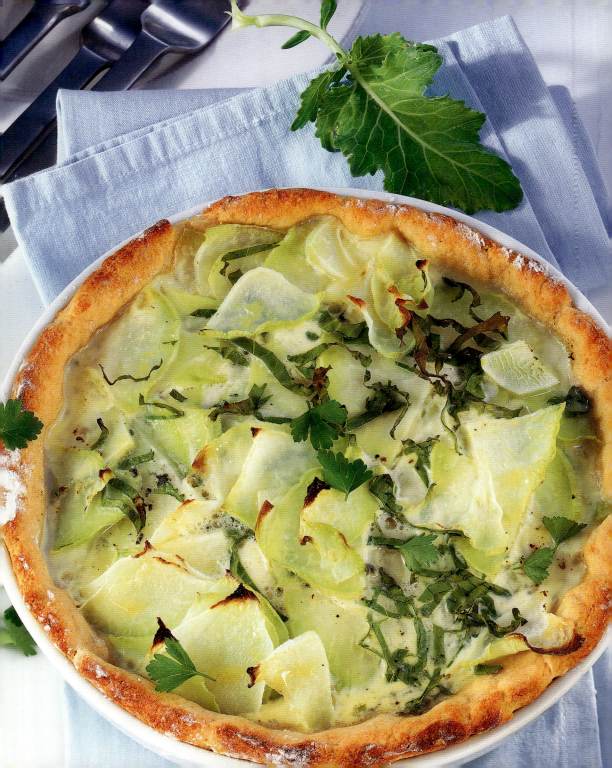

… MAIN COURSES - VEGETARIAN

Lentil Rice with vegetables

SERVES 2

100 g (3⅓ oz) red lentils
80 g (2¾ oz) brown long-grain rice (parboiled)
250 g (8 oz) tomatoes
1 onion
1 garlic clove
2 tbsp rapeseed oil
1 bay leaf
1 clove
1½ tsp mild curry powder
500 ml (16 fl oz/2 cups) vegetable stock
salt, pepper
500 g (1 lb) cauliflower
1 piece fresh ginger (about 1 cm/½ in long)
1 tbsp cashew nuts
2 tbsp freshly chopped coriander (or parsley)
2 tbsp yoghurt (3.5% fat)

PREPARATION: about 1 hour

1. Wash the lentils and the rice and drain well. Briefly dip the tomatoes into boiling water, peel away the skin and chop the flesh. Peel and finely chop the onion and garlic.

2. Heat 1 tablespoon oil in a saucepan and fry the onion and garlic until translucent. Add the bay leaf, clove and curry powder and fry for about 2 minutes. Add the lentils, rice and tomatoes and stir in. Pour in the stock and season generously with salt and pepper. Bring to the boil, cover and simmer over low heat for about 35 minutes. Remove the bay leaf.

3. Meanwhile, trim the cauliflower and separate into florets, then wash and drain. Peel and finely chop the ginger. Heat the remaining oil in a frying pan. Briefly sauté the cauliflower florets and the ginger in the oil, then add 75 ml (2½ fl oz/⅓ cup) water. Cover and cook over medium heat for about 15 minutes or until the cauliflower is just cooked. If necessary, add a little more water during cooking. Season with a little salt.

4. Add the cauliflower mixture to the lentil rice. Turn off the heat and sit for another 5 minutes to draw more flavour. Chop the cashew nuts. Stir the coriander into the lentil rice. Serve with the yoghurt and the cashew nuts.

TIP

Wholegrain rice, also known as brown rice, is ideal for diabetics. It contains plenty of vitamins, minerals and dietary fibre. Another bonus is that its glycemic index is relatively low.

NUTRITIONAL VALUES PER PORTION:
500 Cal • 20 g protein • 17 g fat • 65 g carbohydrate • 14 g dietary fibre • 4 CE

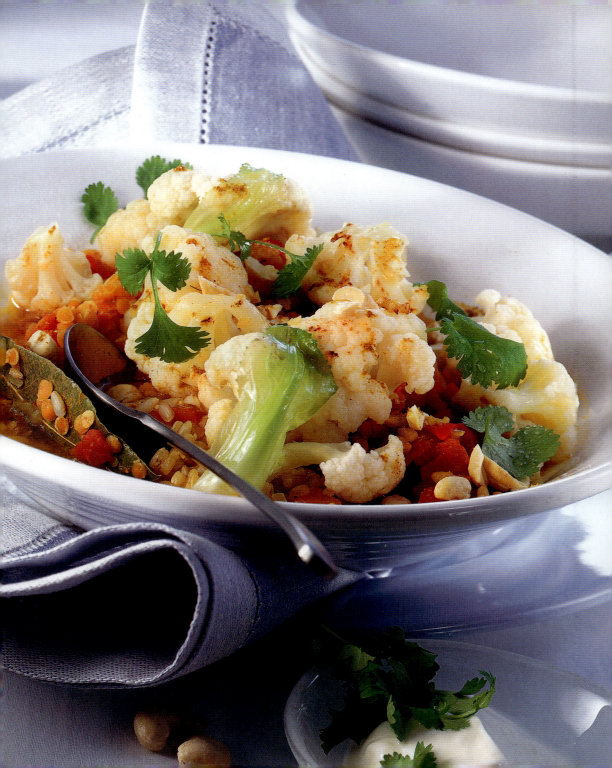

Mackerel baked in foil

SERVES 2
150 g (5 oz) leeks
1 small fennel bulb (about 200 g/6½ oz)
1 small carrot
100 ml (3 fl oz/½ cup) vegetable stock
100 g (3⅓ oz) large mushrooms
½ tsp dried thyme
salt, pepper
4 sprigs parsley
2 mackerel (about 250 g/ 8 oz each)
1 tbsp reduced-fat butter
2 tsp lemon juice
1 tsp oil
400 g (13 oz) small new potatoes
PREPARATION: about 30 mins
COOKING: 30 mins

1. Preheat the oven to 220°C (430°F) /200°C (390°F) fan-forced (middle shelf). Trim and wash or peel the leeks, fennel and carrot, then cut into thin strips (use a julienne cutter if you have one). In a frying pan, bring the stock to the boil and cook the vegetables for about 5 minutes.

2. Brush the mushrooms clean and chop into slices. Add to the vegetables along with the thyme, and season with a little salt and pepper. Wash and shake dry the parsley.

3. Rinse the mackerel under cold water, pat dry with kitchen paper, then fill with the parsley sprigs. Melt the butter in a small frying pan. Remove from the heat and stir in the lemon juice.

4. Brush two large pieces of foil (abut 10 cm/4 in larger than the fish) with the oil. Spread the vegetables with their cooking liquid in the middle of the foil pieces. Place the mackerel on top. Brush with the lemon butter, pepper lightly, then wrap the fish in the foil.

5. Place the mackerel parcels into an ovenproof dish. Bake in the oven for about 30 minutes.

6. Meanwhile, brush clean the potatoes and cook unpeeled in salted water for about 25 minutes. Drain and leave to cool briefly. Serve the mackerel with the potatoes on the side.

TIP
Other types of fish are also suitable for this recipe, for example snapper, bream or trout. Instead of fennel you could also use spring onions along with any other spring vegetables.

TIP
Spoil yourself and indulge in a starter or dessert of your choice with this main course if your individual carbohydrate requirements allow you to do so.

NUTRITIONAL VALUES PER PORTION:
505 Cal • 35 g protein • 21 g fat • 41 g carbohydrate • 11 g dietary fibre • about 2.7 CE

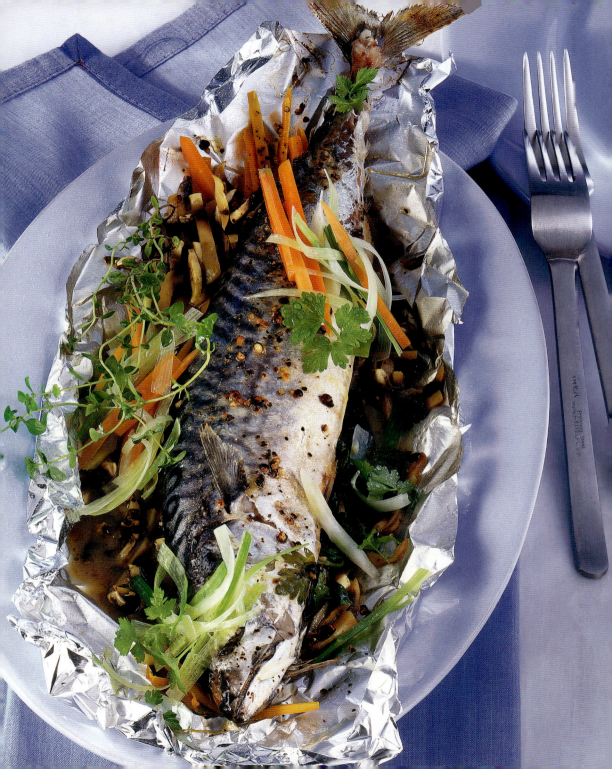

Fish with panfried mushrooms

SERVES 2

400 g (13 oz) potatoes
salt
1 organic lemon
2 shallots
1 garlic clove
300 g (10 oz) mixed mushrooms (e.g. button mushrooms and oyster mushrooms)
2 flathead cutlets (or New Zealand turbot, 200 g/6½ oz each)
pepper
1 tbsp rapeseed oil
½ tsp chopped marjoram
PREPARATION: about 35 mins

1. Wash, peel and quarter the potatoes, then cook in salted water for about 25 minutes. Drain and leave to cool briefly.

2. Grate 2 teaspoons zest from the lemon. Squeeze out the juice. Peel and finely chop the shallots and the garlic. Brush clean then slice the mushrooms.

3. Rinse the fish cutlets under cold water; pat dry with kitchen paper. Season both sides with salt and pepper, then place them in a steamer. Sprinkle with lemon zest. Fill a saucepan about 5 cm (2 in) high with water and add 3 tablespoons lemon juice. Place the steamer in the saucepan, so that it does not sit in the water. Bring the liquid to the boil, cover and steam the fish for about 12 minutes.

4. Heat the oil in a non-stick pan and fry the shallots, garlic, mushrooms and marjoram, stirring constantly, until golden. Season with salt and pepper. Serve the fish cutlets with the potatoes and the mushrooms.

TIP
The Chicory & Grape Salad (see page 40) goes well as an entrée.

NUTRITIONAL VALUES PER PORTION:
425 Cal • 8 g protein • 10 g fat • 32 g carbohydrate • 6 g dietary fibre • 2 CE

Cod with leek and tomatoes

SERVES 2

1 small tin peeled tomatoes (400 g/13 oz)
1 bunch parsley
500 g (1 lb) leeks
1 tbsp oil
salt, pepper
120 g (4 oz) brown long-grain rice (parboiled)
300 g (10 oz) cod fillet
1 tbsp lemon juice
PREPARATION: about 30 mins
COOKING: 25 MINS

1. Drain the tomatoes, reserving the juice. Rinse and shake dry the parsley, then finely chop. Trim the leeks, slice open lengthways and thoroughly wash. Cut into 1 cm (½ in) slices. Heat the oil in a non-stick pan and sauté the leek slices for about 3 minutes. Roughly chop and add the tomatoes. Stir in 4 tablespoons tomato juice and half the parsley. Season with salt and pepper to taste.

2. Cook the rice as per packet instructions. Preheat the oven to 200°C (390°F) /180°C (355°F) fan-forced (bottom shelf), removing the oven rack. Rinse the cod under cold water, pat dry with kitchen paper and season with lemon juice, salt and pepper. Use an oven bag and close one end according to instructions. Arrange the vegetable mixture in the bag; place the fish on top.

3. Close the foil end. Pierce the oven bag once or twice in the top and place on the cold oven rack. Cook the fish in the oven for about 25 minutes. Sprinkle with the remaining parsley. Serve the cod with the rice and vegetables.

NUTRITIONAL VALUES PER PORTION:
435 Cal • 36 g protein • 7 g fat • 55 g carbohydrate • 5 g dietary fibre • about 3.3 CE

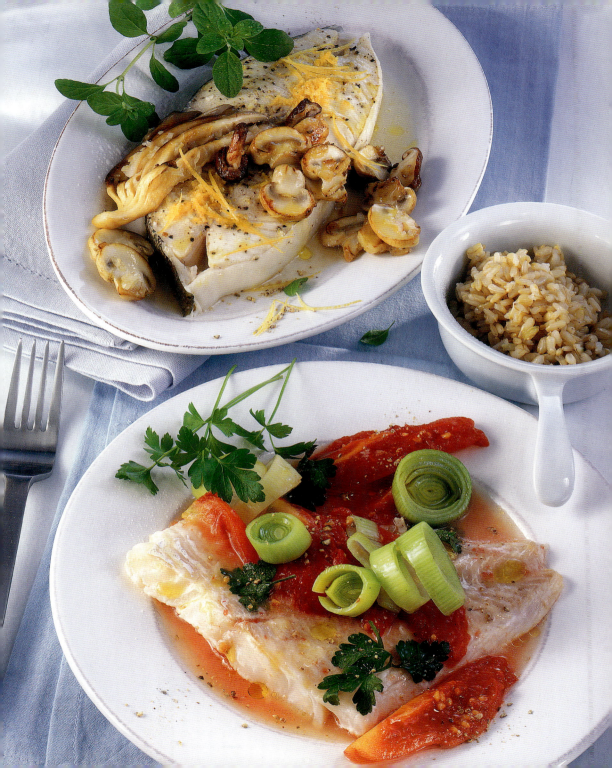

Fish Fillets in a sesame crust

SERVES 2

125 g (4 oz) small green lentils (Puy lentils)

300 ml (10 fl oz/1¼ cups) vegetable stock

1 small ripe mango (about 200 g/6½ oz)

1 pinch cayenne pepper (or 1 tbsp hot chilli sauce)

1¼ tbsp lemon juice

salt, pepper

1 tsp olive oil

300 g (10 oz) blue-eyed cod fillet (or snapper filet)

1 egg white

2½ tbsp unhulled sesame seeds

2 tbsp wholemeal breadcrumbs

1 tbsp wholemeal flour

1 small carrot

2 spring onions

4 chicory leaves

1 piece fresh ginger root (about 1 cm/½ in long)

2½ tbsp rapeseed oil

½ tsp balsamic vinegar

PREPARATION: about 1 hr

1. Rinse the lentils under cold water, place in a saucepan with the stock and bring to the boil. Cover and simmer over low heat for about 45 minutes. Peel the mango. Cut the flesh from the stone, roughly chop and then purée using a hand-held blender. Season with cayenne pepper, ¼ tablespoon lemon juice, salt and pepper and stir in the olive oil. Cover the mango sauce and set aside at room temperature.

2. Rinse the fish under cold water, pat dry with kitchen paper and cut into 4 pieces. Drizzle with ½ tablespoon lemon juice and season on both sides with salt and pepper. Whisk the egg white. Combine the sesame seeds and breadcrumbs. Dust the fish on both sides with flour, turn first in the egg white, then in the sesame seed mixture. Press the crust well into the fish flesh. Cover the fish and place in the fridge to chill.

3. Meanwhile trim, peel and finely dice the carrot. Trim, wash and finely chop the spring onions. Rinse the chicory leaves under cold water and shake dry. Peel and finely grate the ginger. Drain the lentils.

4. In a saucepan heat ½ tablespoon oil. Add the carrots, half the spring onions and the ginger and sauté until the onions are translucent. Stir in the lentils and briefly heat through. Season with salt, pepper and balsamic vinegar. Turn off the heat, cover and leave to draw more flavour.

5. Heat the remaining oil in a non-stick frying pan and fry the fish pieces for about 6 minutes until golden, turning them once. Drizzle the fish with the remaining lemon juice. Stir the remaining spring onions into the mango sauce. On each serving plate, place half the fish and 2 chicory leaves. Pile the lentil mixture into the chicory "boats". Serve with the mango sauce.

NUTRITIONAL VALUES PER PORTION:
685 Cal • 51 g protein • 26 g fat • 61 g carbohydrate • 14 g dietary fibre • 4 CE

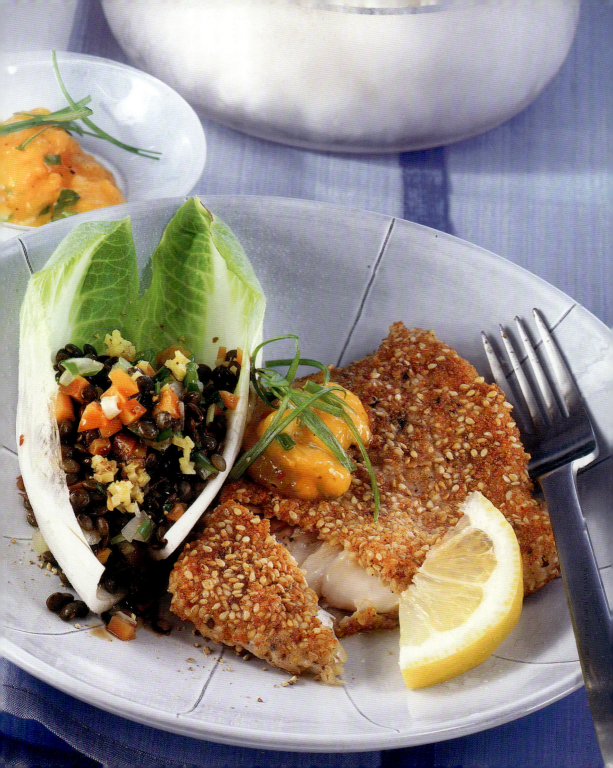

Barramundi in an olive and caper sauce

SERVES 2

50 g (1⅔ oz) pitted black olives
½ tsp Dijon mustard
salt, pepper
2 tbsp lemon juice
1 pinch grated lemon zest
3 tbsp olive oil
2 tbsp capers
1 tbsp chopped parsley
½ tsp fennel seeds
400 g (13 oz) barramundi fillet
150 g (5 oz) wholemeal pasta,
  e.g. farfalle
75 ml (2½ oz/⅓ cup) fish stock (or vegetable stock)

PREPARATION: about 25 mins

1. Finely chop the olives. Whisk together the mustard, salt, pepper, lemon juice and zest. Add the oil, capers, parsley and olives.

2. Lightly crush the fennel seeds in a mortar and pestle. Rinse the fish under cold water, pat dry with kitchen paper and cut into 2 cm (¾ in) pieces. Season the fish with salt, pepper and fennel. Cook the pasta as per the packet instructions in salt water until al dente (firm to the bite).

3. Meanwhile heat the stock, add the fish, cover and sauté in the stock for about 5 minutes.

4. Drain the pasta, then stir in the fish along with all the cooking liquid. Arrange on plates and drizzle with the olive and caper sauce. A green salad with a yoghurt and herb dressing would make for a tasty accompaniment.

NUTRITIONAL VALUES PER PORTION:
640 Cal • 48 g protein • 27 g fat • 52 g carbohydrate • 6 g dietary fibre • about 3.3 CE

Fish Kebabs with lemon sauce

SERVES 2

300 g (10 oz) fish fillet
  (e.g. blue-eyed cod, barramundi or ocean trout)
salt
250 g (8 oz) broccoli
100 g (3⅓ oz) small cherry tomatoes
½ organic lemon
1 bunch parsley
120 g (4 oz) Basmati rice
1 tbsp olive oil
coarsely ground pepper
75 ml (2½ oz/⅓ cup) vegetable stock

PREPARATION: about 35 mins

1. Rinse fish under cold water, pat dry with kitchen paper and cut into 3 cm (1¼ in) dice. Season with salt. Trim the broccoli, separate into florets and blanch in boiling salted water for 3 minutes. Rinse under cold water and drain; season with salt. Wash the tomatoes.

2. Thread the fish cubes, broccoli florets and tomatoes onto four kebab skewers. Finely grate the zest of the lemon half and squeeze out the juice. Wash, shake dry and finely chop the parsley. Cook the rice as per the packet instructions.

3. Heat the oil in a non-stick pan. Stir in 2 tablespoons lemon juice and a little coarsely ground pepper. Place the fish kebabs into the pan and fry both sides for 3 minutes. Add the stock and the lemon zest. Cook for a further 3–4 minutes.

4. Stir the chopped pasley into the cooked rice. Arrange the fish kebabs with the herbed rice on serving plates. Check and adjust the seasoning in the pan with salt, pepper and lemon juice, then drizzle over the fish kebabs.

NUTRITIONAL VALUES PER PORTION:
410 Cal • 35 g protein • 7 g fat • 50 g carbohydrate • 4 g dietary fibre • about 3.3 CE

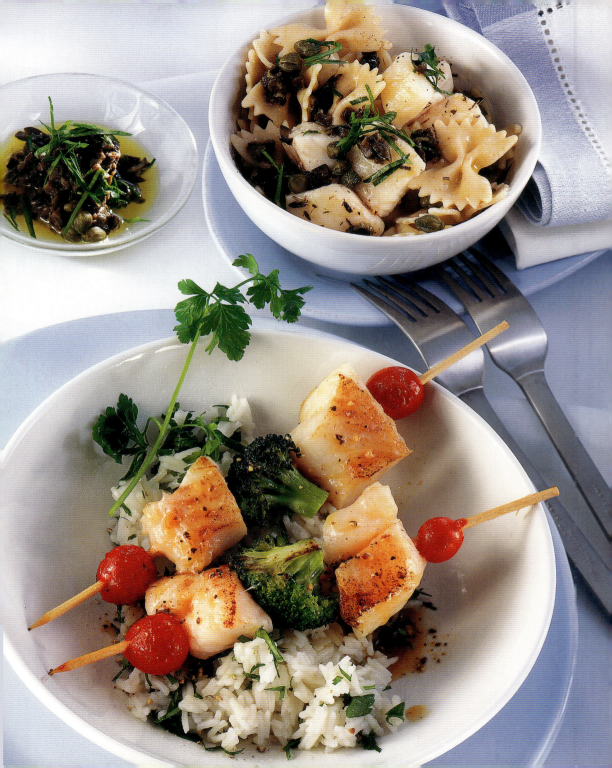

Ocean Perch Ragout

SERVES 2

400 g (13 oz) ocean perch fillet

salt, pepper

2 tbsp lemon juice

200 ml (7 fl oz/¾ cup) vegetable stock

1 small onion

1 bay leaf

1 tsp mustard seeds (or ½ tsp hot mustard)

120 g (4 oz) brown long-grain rice (parboiled)

100 g (3⅓ oz) celeriac

1 small red capsicum (pepper)

1 organic orange

½ bunch flat-leaf parsley

50 g (1⅔ oz) sour cream

PREPARATION: about 45 mins

1. Rinse the fish under cold water and pat dry with kitchen paper. Season with salt and pepper and drizzle with 1 tablespoon lemon juice. In a shallow saucepan, bring the stock to the boil. Peel the onion and cut into eighths. Add to the stock, with the bay leaf, mustard seeds and a little salt.

2. Place the fish in the stock. Turn off the heat, cover and set aside for 15–20 minutes to draw flavour. Meanwhile cook the rice as per the packet instructions.

3. Peel and grate the celeriac. Trim, wash and finely chop the capsicum. Lift the fish out of the cooking liquid. Pass the liquid through a sieve and return to the saucepan. Cook the vegetables in the liquid for about 10 minutes.

4. Peel the orange and cut the fillets from between the membranes, catching the juice. Wash, shake dry and chop the parsley, reserving a few leaves. Cut the fish into bite-sized pieces.

5. Set aside 2 tablespoons vegetables, purée the rest with a little cooking liquid. Stir in the cream and heat through without boiling. Add the orange juice and enough cooking liquid to make a smooth sauce. Add the fish, the reserved vegetables, and the orange fillets and briefly heat through. Season the ragout with salt, pepper and lemon juice. Serve with the rice.

TIP

Instead of ocean perch you can use any other fish fillet of your choice. Make sure you choose a fish with firm flesh and which is light in colour.

NUTRITIONAL VALUES PER PORTION:
465 Cal • 43 g protein • 6 g fat • 55 g carbohydrate • 7 g dietary fibre • about 3.7 CE

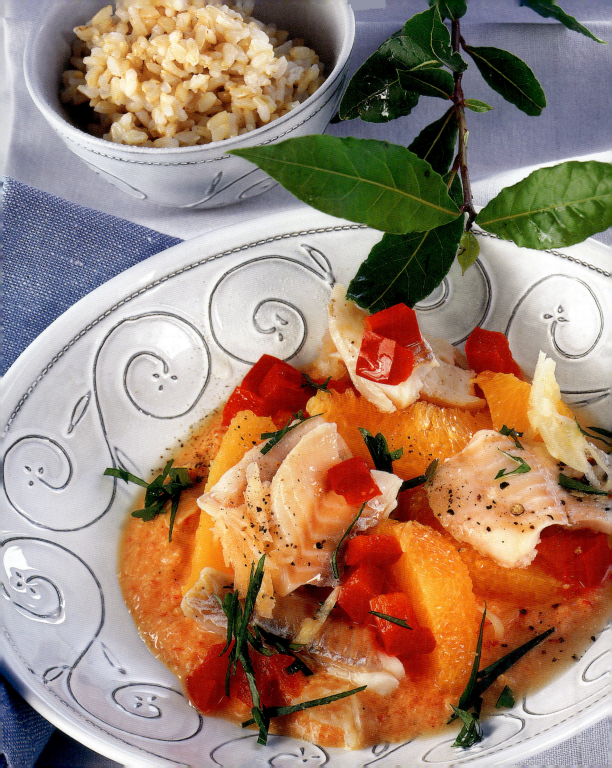

Capsicum Barley with prawns

SERVES 2

200 g (6½ oz) frozen shelled prawns
1 red, 1 yellow and 1 green capsicum (pepper, about 600 g/1 lb 3 oz)
1 organic lemon
1 garlic clove
2 tbsp olive oil
120 g (4 oz) pearl barley
400 ml (14 fl oz/1¾ cups) fish stock (or vegetable stock)
salt, pepper
1 tbsp parsley leaves

PREPARATION: about 40 mins

1. Leave the prawns to defrost slightly. Meanwhile trim and wash the capsicums, then finely chop. Finely grate the zest of half the lemon. Peel and finely dice the garlic.

2. Heat the oil in a shallow saucepan, add the garlic and fry until translucent. Add the barley and the capsicum and briefly cook with the garlic. Add the stock and stir in the lemon zest. Season to taste with salt and pepper. Briefly bring everything to the boil, then cover the saucepan and simmer over low heat for about 20 minutes.

3. Wash the prawns and place on top of the barley. Simmer for a further 15 minutes. Check and adjust the seasoning. Cut the remaining lemon half into wedges. Arrange the barley and prawn mixture on serving plates. Garnish with parsley leaves and lemon wedges.

NUTRITIONAL VALUES PER PORTION:
470 Cal • 27 g protein • 15 g fat • 55 g carbohydrate • 10 g dietary fibre • about 3.7 CE

Ling Fillet in a cheese & vegetable crust

SERVES 2

2 ling fillets (about 200 g/6½ oz each)
salt, pepper
2 tbsp olive oil
500 g (1 lb) zucchini (courgette)
1 bunch spring onions
1 garlic clove
1 tsp tomato paste
1 tsp dried thyme
100 ml (3 fl oz/½ cup) vegetable stock
120 g (4 oz) Basmati rice
100 g (3⅓ oz) mozzarella

PREPARATION: about 35 mins

1. Preheat the oven to 220°C (430°F) /200°C (390°F) fan-forced (middle shelf). Rinse the fish under cold water, pat dry with kitchen paper and season with salt and pepper. Thinly brush an ovenproof dish with oil. Place the fish fillets side by side in the dish.

2. Wash and trim the vegetables. Finely chop the zucchini; slice the spring onions. Heat the remaining oil in a non-stick pan, add the zucchini and spring onions and fry for about 5 minutes. Peel and crush the garlic and add to the pan. Stir in the tomato paste and thyme. Cook for a short time. Pour in the stock, then season the vegetables with salt and pepper and remove from the heat.

3. Cook the rice as per the packet instructions. Drain the mozzarella well, roughly grate and stir into the vegetables. Spread the vegetable and mozzarella mixture on top of the fish. Cook in the oven for about 15 minutes. Serve the fish with the rice.

NUTRITIONAL VALUES PER PORTION:
640 Cal • 54 g protein • 23 g fat • 63 g carbohydrate • 4 g dietary fibre • about 4 CE

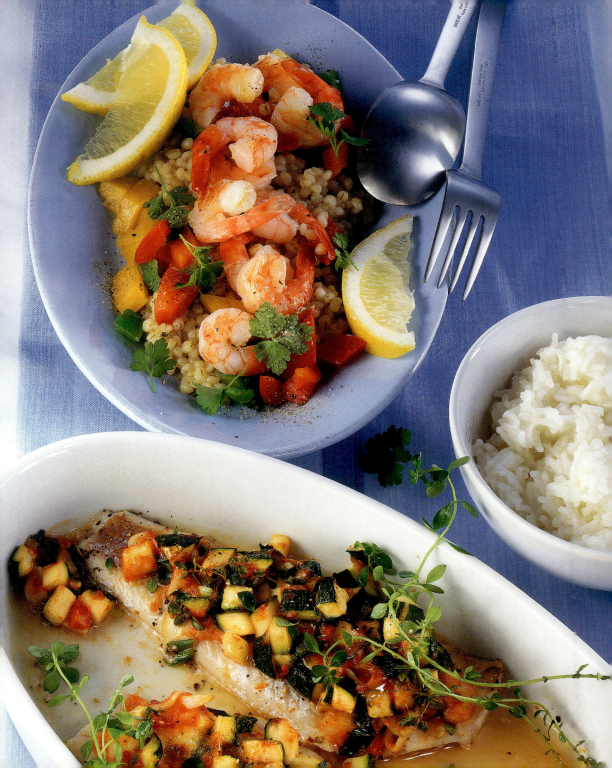

Salmon on Waldorf salad

SERVES 2

4 salmon fillets, skinned (about 80 g/2¾ oz each)
salt
2 tsp reduced-fat butter
150 g (5 oz) celeriac
3 tbsp lemon juice
2 celery sticks
400 g (13 oz) small new potatoes
1 tbsp walnuts
2 tbsp sour cream
1 small red apple
pepper

PREPARATION: about 45 mins

1. Rinse the fish under cold water, pat dry with kitchen paper and season with salt. Melt the butter and thinly brush a plate with it. Place the fish fillets next to each other on the plate and brush with the remaining butter. Cover with cling film and pull tightly across the fish.

2. Preheat the oven to 80°C (175°F) /60°C (140°F) fan-forced (middle shelf). Peel the celeriac and cut first into slices, then into short sticks. Bring to the boil 250 ml (8 fl oz/1 cup) water with a little salt and lemon juice. Blanch the celeriac for 7 minutes.

3. Wash, trim and then thinly slice the celery. Reserve the tender celery greens. Add the celery to the celeriac and blanch for a further 2 minutes. Remove from the heat.

4. Wash the potatoes and cook (unpeeled) in salted water for about 20 minutes until soft. Cook the fish fillets in the oven for about 20 minutes.

5. Finely chop the celery greens and roughly chop the walnuts. Stir the sour cream into the vegetables and heat through again. Wash, quarter and core the apple, then cut into short sticks. Stir the apple into the vegetables along with the walnuts. Season with a little salt, pepper and lemon juice to taste.

6. Peel the skin off the potatoes and combine with the chopped celery greens. Arrange the fish, vegetables and potatoes on hot serving plates.

> **TIP**
> Salmon stays wonderfully moist and aromatic if cooked gently as per this recipe. It is important that the oven temperature is between 80°C (175°F) and a maximum of 85°C (185°F) or 55°C (130°F)-60°C (140°F) fan-forced). You can check this with an oven thermometer (available in household and department stores). If you have a gas oven, use the lowest setting and leave the oven door slightly ajar.

NUTRITIONAL VALUES PER PORTION:
600 Cal • 39 g protein • 31 g fat • 40 g carbohydrate • 9 g dietary fibre • about 2.7 CE

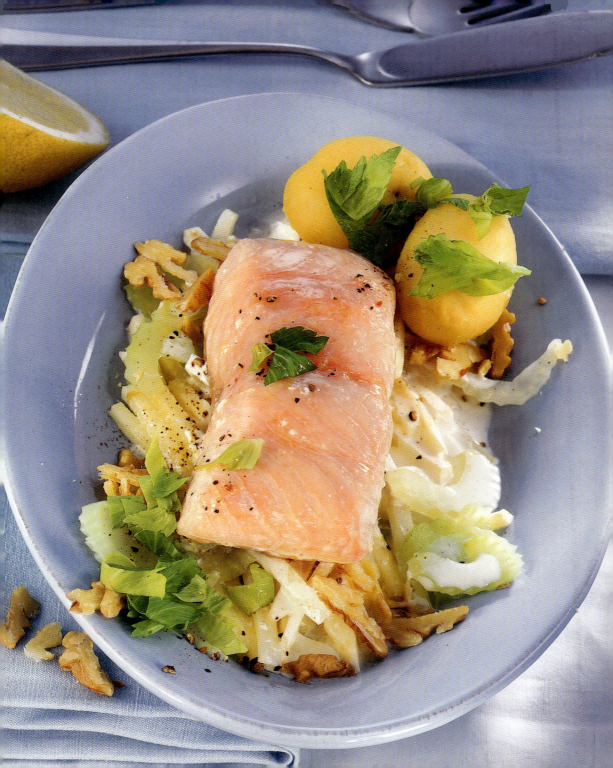

Barramundi & Vegetables

SERVES 2

150 g (5 oz) celeriac
1 yellow capsicum (pepper)
150 g (5 oz) zucchini (courgette)
4 spring onions
1 tbsp rapeseed oil
1 tsp dried thyme
salt, pepper
300 g (10 oz) barramundi fillet (or any other fish fillet)
100 ml (3 fl oz/½ cup) vegetable stock
1 tbsp lemon juice
120 g (4 oz) Basmati rice
3 tbsp cream

PREPARATION: about 35 mins

1. Trim, peel and chop the celeriac. Trim, wash and chop the capsicum. Wash and trim the zucchini and the spring onions. Slice the zucchini and cut the spring onions diagonally into short lengths. Heat the oil in a non-stick frying pan and sauté the vegetables for about 5 minutes. Season with the thyme, salt and pepper, and push the vegetables to the edges of the frying pan.

2. Rinse the fish under cold water, pat dry with kitchen paper and roughly chop. Season with salt and pepper and place in the middle of the pan. Pour over the stock and the lemon juice. Cover and cook over low heat for about 12 minutes. Meanwhile, cook the Basmati rice as per the packet instructions.

3. Combine the fish and the vegetables. Drizzle over the cream and heat for another 1–2 minutes. Serve the fish and vegetables with the rice.

NUTRITIONAL VALUES PER PORTION:
505 Cal • 37 g protein • 16 g fat • 52 g carbohydrate • 7 g dietary fibre • about 3.3 CE

Fish Osso Buco

SERVES 2

2 cod cutlets (200 g/6½ oz each)
2 tsp wholemeal flour
salt, pepper
1 onion
100 g (3/3 oz) carrots
200 g (6½ oz) leeks
1 tbsp olive oil
50 ml (2 fl oz/¼ cup) white wine (or vegetable stock)
200 ml (7 fl oz/¾ cup) vegetable stock
1 sprig thyme
120 g (4 oz) wholegrain long-grain rice (parboiled)
½ bunch parsley
1 organic lemon
1 garlic clove

PREPARATION: about 40 mins

1. Rinse the fish cutlets under cold water; pat dry with kitchen paper. Add a little salt and pepper to the flour. Turn the cutlets in the seasoned flour. Peel and finely chop the onion and the carrots. Trim the leeks and wash, then cut into strips.

2. Heat the oil and fry the fish cutlets on both sides for about 2 minutes, then remove. Add the onion, carrots and leeks and sauté for about 5 minutes in the frying liquid. Season with a little salt and pepper. Pour in the wine and stock, then add the thyme. Bring to the boil, then reduce the heat. Add the fish cutlets to the vegetables, cover and simmer over low heat for about 20 minutes.

3. Meanwhile, cook the rice as per the packet instructions. Wash and shake dry the parsley, then finely chop. Grate 2 teaspoons zest from the lemon. Peel and finely chop the garlic. Combine the parsley with the zest and the garlic.

4. Arrange the fish cutlets with the vegetables and the cooking liquid. Sprinkle with the parsley and lemon mixture. Serve the osso buco with the rice.

NUTRITIONAL VALUES PER PORTION:
490 Cal • 42 g protein • 9 g fat • 55 g carbohydrate • 6 g dietary fibre • about 3.7 CE

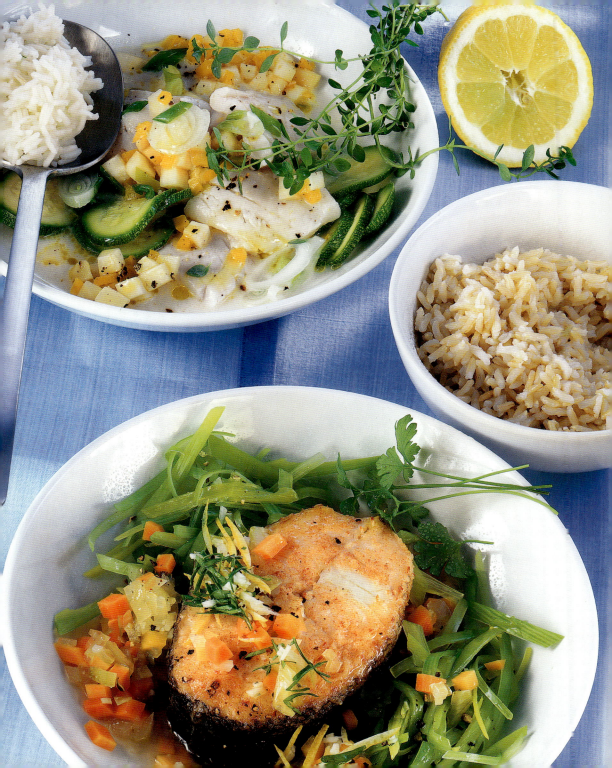

Creole Chicken Casserole

SERVES 2

250 g (8 oz) chicken breast fillet
½ tsp allspice (or 2 cloves)
salt, pepper
2½ tbsp lemon juice
1 yellow capsicum (pepper)
300 g (10 oz) zucchini (courgette)
250 g (8 oz) sweet potato
½ red chilli
1 onion
1 garlic clove
1 tbsp olive oil
½ tsp dried thyme
250 ml (8 fl oz/1 cup) chicken stock (or vegetable stock)
2 lemon slices
60 g (2 oz) wholemeal baguette

PREPARATION: about 45 mins

1. Cut the chicken into 2 cm (¾ in) pieces, then season with half the allspice, salt, pepper and 1 tablespoon lemon juice.

2. Quarter the capsicum lengthways, trim and rinse, then cut crossways into strips. Wash, trim and halve the zucchini lengthways, then cut into 1 cm (½ in) slices. Wash and peel the sweet potato and cut into 1.5 cm (⅔ in) dice. Drizzle the capsicum, zucchini and sweet potatoes with 1 tablespoon lemon juice. Trim and wash the chilli, then cut into rings. Peel and dice the onion and garlic.

3. Heat the oil in a saucepan and fry the chicken breasts on both sides for 3 minutes. Add the onion and garlic and briefly fry. Add the vegetables and chilli. Season with the salt, thyme and remaining allspice. Pour in the stock.

4. Cover and cook over medium heat for about 25 minutes. Season with the remaining lemon juice. Garnish with the lemon slices and serve with the baguette.

TIP

Sweet potatoes have a lower glycemic index than other potatoes. However, if you prefer, you can substitute floury potatoes instead.

TIP

Chillies add more than heat to this dish – they can also improve your circulation. If you don't like your food too hot, simply halve the chilli lengthways and remove the seeds. It's best to wear rubber gloves when handling chilli and do not rub your eyes or other sensitive parts with your fingers. If you don't like hot food at all, just leave out the chilli altogether.

NUTRITIONAL VALUES PER PORTION:
470 Cal • 37 g protein • 10 g fat • 55 g carbohydrate • 11 g dietary fibre • about 3.3 CE

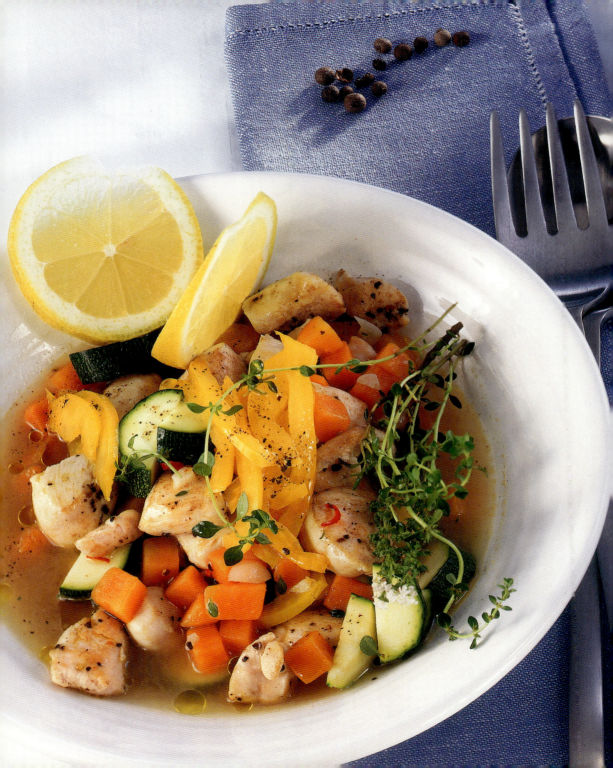

Filled Turkey Rolls

SERVES 2

½ bunch parsley
4 sprigs basil
1 garlic clove
10 g (½ oz) walnuts
2 tbsp grated Parmesan
2 tsp olive oil
2 turkey escalopes (120 g/4 oz each)
salt, pepper
3 celery sticks
1 onion
200 g (6½ oz) chopped tomatoes (tinned)
2 bay leaves
120 g (4 oz) fettucine (made from durum wheat)

PREPARATION: about 30 mins
COOKING: 35 mins

1. Wash and shake dry the herbs. Peel and roughly chop the garlic. Purée the herbs, garlic, nuts, Parmesan and oil in a blender.

2. Preheat the oven to 200°C (390°F) / 180°C (355°F) fan-forced (middle shelf) and remove the oven rack. Flatten the escalopes and season them with salt and pepper. Spread the herb and nut paste on the escalopes, then roll them up and tie into rolls with kitchen string.

3. Trim, wash and dice the celery. Season with salt and pepper. Set the tender celery greens aside. Peel and finely chop the onion. Close one end of an oven bag as per packet instructions. Fill with the celery, onion, tomatoes, bay leaves and turkey rolls.

4. Close the other end of the bag well, and pierce once or twice on top. Place the bag on the cold rack, then cook in the oven for about 35 minutes. Cook the pasta as per the packet instructions in salted water until al dente (firm to the bite), then drain. Arrange turkey rolls and vegetables on plates with the pasta, sprinkle with the celery greens and serve immediately.

NUTRITIONAL VALUES PER PORTION:
500 Cal • 44 g protein • 13 g fat • 52 g carbohydrate • 3 g dietary fibre • about 3.3 CE

Curried Turkey Strips

SERVES 2

120 g (4 oz) long-grain rice (parboiled)
200 g (6½ oz) turkey breast fillet
1 bunch spring onions
3 dried apricots
2 tbsp rapeseed oil
salt, pepper
1 tsp curry powder
150 g (5 oz) frozen peas
125 ml (4 fl oz/½ cup) chicken stock
2 tbsp sour cream

PREPARATION: about 30 mins

1. Cook the rice as per the packet instructions. Rinse the turkey breast under cold water, pat dry and cut across the fibre into 4 cm (1½ in) strips. Trim and wash the spring onions; slice diagonally into 3 cm (1¼ in) lengths. Cut the apricots into strips.

2. In a frying pan heat 1 tablespoon oil and fry the turkey on both sides for 2–3 minutes. Season with salt and pepper and take out of the pan. Add the remaining oil and briefly fry the spring onions. Sprinkle with ½ teaspoon curry powder.

3. Add the peas, apricots and stock to the spring onions. Quickly bring to the boil, cover and simmer for 5 minutes. Stir in the turkey strips and heat through for about 1 minute. Stir in the sour cream and season with the remaining curry powder, salt and pepper to taste. Serve with the rice.

NUTRITIONAL VALUES PER PORTION:
530 Cal • 34 g protein • 18 g fat • 61 g carbohydrate • 3 g dietary fibre • 4 CE

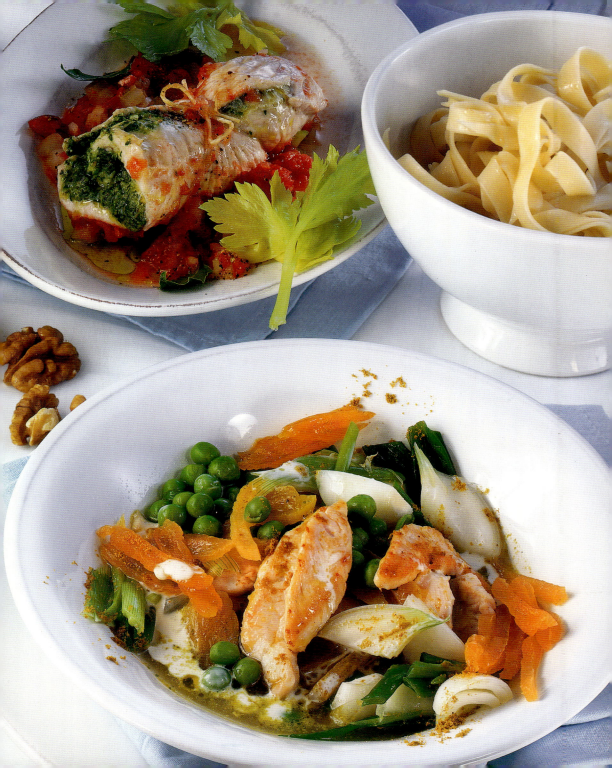

Chicken Breast with pineapple

SERVES 2

250 g (8 oz) chicken breast fillet
4 tbsp teriyaki sauce for meat (or light soy sauce)
120 g (4 oz) long-grain rice (parboiled)
1 red capsicum (pepper)
1 carrot
1 small Chinese cabbage (about 400 g/13 oz)
1 tbsp rapeseed oil
100 g (3⅓ oz) fresh pineapple (or unsweetened tinned pineapple pieces)
salt, pepper

PREPARATION: about 40 mins

1. Briefly rinse the chicken breasts, pat dry and cut across the fibre into pieces. Combine with the teriyaki sauce, cover and place in the fridge for 20 minutes to marinate.

2. Cook the rice as per the packet instructions. Trim and wash the capsicum, then cut into chunks. Trim, peel and thinly slice the carrot. Trim and wash the Chinese cabbage, then cut into strips.

3. Heat the oil in a frying pan and briefly cook the chicken including the marinade over high heat, stirring constantly. Add the capsicum and carrot and fry for 3 minutes.

4. Stir in the Chinese cabbage and cook for a further 5 minutes, stirring constantly, until the chicken is cooked. Add a little water if needed. Cut the pineapple into small chunks, add and heat through. Season with salt and pepper to taste. Serve with the rice.

NUTRITIONAL VALUES PER PORTION:
425 Cal • 37 g protein • 8 g fat • 58 g carbohydrate • 10 g dietary fibre • 4 CE

Duck Breast with broccoli and nuts

SERVES 2

1 small duck breast fillet (about 250 g/8 oz)
400 g (13 oz) broccoli
salt
110 g (4 oz) Basmati rice
1 onion
1 garlic clove
1 piece fresh ginger (about 1 cm/½ in long)
50 ml (2 fl oz/¼ cup) chicken stock
3 tbsp light soy sauce
2 tbsp vegetable oil
2 tbsp unsalted cashew nuts
pepper
2 tbsp desiccated coconut

PREPARATION: about 30 mins

1. Skin the duck breast, then cut the flesh into 1 cm (½ in) strips. Trim and wash the broccoli, separate into florets. Peel and finely chop the broccoli stems. Blanch the stems for 2 minutes in boiling salted water, adding the florets for the second minute. Rinse the broccoli under cold water and drain well.

2. Cook the rice as per the packet instructions. Meanwhile, peel the onion, cut into eighths, then separate the layers. Peel and finely chop the garlic and the ginger. Stir together the stock and the soy sauce.

3. Heat the oil in a frying pan and briefly roast the cashew nuts, then remove. Fry the duck breast in the pan briefly over high heat, stirring constantly. Remove from the pan.

4. In the same pan, fry the broccoli, onion, garlic and ginger over high heat, stirring constantly. Season with salt. After a few minutes pour in the stock mixture. Stir in the duck breast and the cashew nuts. Heat through, then season with salt and pepper. Stir the coconut into the rice and serve with the duck breast.

NUTRITIONAL VALUES PER PORTION:
700 Cal • 37 g protein • 40 g fat • 52 g carbohydrate • 8 g dietary fibre • about 3.3 CE

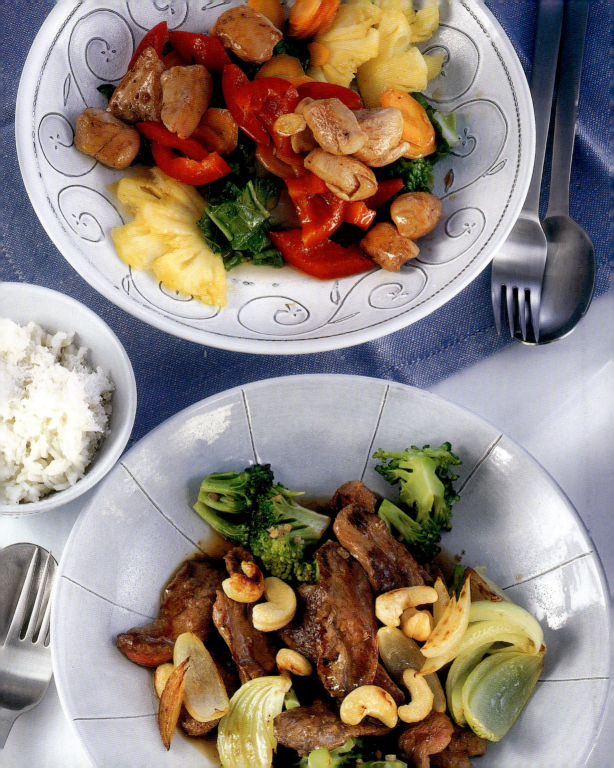

Lemon Chicken

SERVES 2
4 small chicken legs
1 organic lemon
1 sprig rosemary
2 tsp olive oil
salt, pepper
300 g (10 oz) celeriac
2 garlic cloves
400 g (13 oz) potatoes
PREPARATION: about 25 mins
COOKING: about 45 mins

1. Preheat the oven to 200°C (390°F) /180°C (355°F) fan-forced (middle shelf). Remove the oven rack. Skin the chicken legs, wash and pat dry with kitchen paper. Halve each one in the joint. Finely grate the zest of the lemon. Peel the lemon and cut the fillets out between the membranes, catching the juice.

2. Wash and shake dry the rosemary, reserving 1 teaspoon needles and chop the rest very finely. Combine the grated zest, the chopped rosemary, the oil and a little salt and pepper, then rub the chicken legs with the mixture.

3. Peel and finely chop the celeriac. Season with salt and pepper. Peel the garlic. Close one end of an oven bag as per the packet instructions. Place the chicken legs, celeriac, garlic, lemon wedges, reserved lemon juice and remaining rosemary into the oven bag.

4. Firmly close the end of the bag. Pierce the oven bag once or twice at the top and place on the rack. Put the cold rack into the centre of the oven and place a dripping tray underneath. Roast in the oven for about 45 minutes until golden. Meanwhile, wash, peel and quarter the potatoes and cook in salted water for about 25 minutes. Serve with the chicken.

NUTRITIONAL VALUES PER PORTION:
445 Cal • 56 g protein • 8 g fat • 34 g carbohydrate • 8 g dietary fibre • 2 CE

Oven-baked Turkey Drumstick

SERVES 2
1 turkey drumstick (about 400 g/13 oz)
salt, pepper
½ tsp sweet paprika
3 onions
1-2 garlic cloves
2 leeks
½ celeriac
350 g (11½ oz) waxy potatoes
½ tsp dried thyme
200 ml (7 fl oz/¾ cup) chicken stock
PREPARATION: about 20 mins
COOKING: 1 hr

1. Briefly rinse the turkey drumstick and pat it dry. Combine a little salt, pepper and sweet paprika; rub all over the turkey leg. Peel and chop the onions and the garlic. Trim, wash and chop the leeks. Peel and chop the celeriac. Wash, peel and dice the potatoes.

2. Place the vegetables and potatoes in a big roasting pan. Sprinkle with thyme. Place the turkey leg on top. Pour over the stock. Cover the pan and place in the cold oven (bottom shelf). Heat the oven to 200°C (390°F) /180°C (355°F) fan-forced. Cook for 45 minutes, then remove the lid and cook for a further 10–15 minutes, letting it brown a little; turn over the meat occasionally.

3. Remove the turkey and cut the flesh from the bones. Season the potato and vegetable mixture with salt and pepper. Serve with the turkey.

TIP
Serve Hummus (see page 30) as an entrée with this dish, along with 2 slices wholemeal toast (about 30 g/1 oz each). This is the equivalent of about 1.3 CE per person.

NUTRITIONAL VALUES PER PORTION:
375 Cal • 31 g protein • 6 g fat • 25 g carbohydrate • 4 g dietary fibre • about 1.7 CE

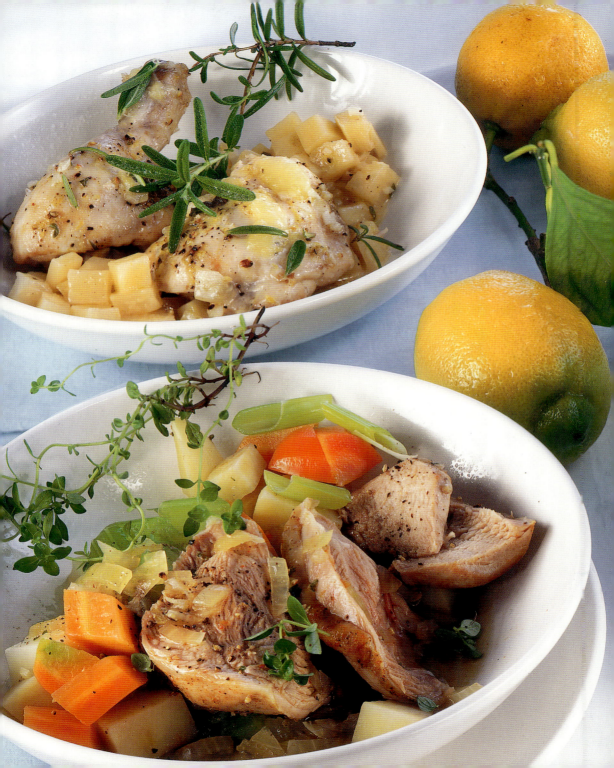

Lasagne with meat & vegetables

SERVES 2

125 g (4 oz) carrots
1 small leek (about 125 g/4 oz)
150 g (5 oz) celery
1 onion
1 garlic clove
1 small sprig rosemary
4 tbsp olive oil
100 g (3⅓ oz) lean beef mince
2 tbsp tomato paste
¼ tsp dried thyme
½ tsp dried oregano
salt, pepper
350 ml (12 fl oz/1½ cups) vegetable stock
2½ tbsp wholemeal flour
250 ml (8 fl oz/1 cup) low-fat milk (1.5% fat)
50 g (1⅔oz) grated Parmesan
1 pinch freshly grated nutmeg
6 sheets wholemeal lasagne (100 g/3⅓ oz)

PREPARATION: about 45 mins
BAKING: about 30 mins

1. Trim, wash and finely dice the carrots, leek and celery. Peel and finely chop the onion and the garlic. Wash and pat dry the rosemary, strip off the needles and chop finely.

2. In a saucepan, heat 1 tablespoon oil and fry the minced meat for about 5 minutes until browned. Add the onion, garlic and vegetables and fry for 3 minutes. Stir in the tomato paste. Season with rosemary, thyme, oregano, salt and pepper. Pour in 250 ml (8 fl oz/1 cup) stock. Cover and simmer the minced meat sauce for about 20 minutes over low heat, stirring occasionally.

3. Meanwhile heat 2 tablespoons oil in a saucepan to make the béchamel sauce. Briefly fry the flour in the oil. Take the saucepan off the heat and stir in the milk and remaining stock. Heat through the sauce, stirring constantly and simmer for about 5 minutes. Stir in 10 g (½ oz) Parmesan. Season the béchamel sauce with salt, pepper and nutmeg to taste.

4. Preheat the oven to 200°C (390°F) /180°C (355°F) fan-forced (middle shelf). Brush a small, shallow ovenproof dish with oil. Put a little of the meat sauce into the dish. Fill the dish with lasagne sheets, meat sauce and béchamel sauce, finishing with the béchamel. Sprinkle with the remaining Parmesan and drizzle with 1 tablespoon oil. Bake the lasagne in the oven for about 30 minutes.

VARIATION

If you prefer a vegetarian lasagne, just leave out the minced meat and increase the amount of carrots, leek and celery by about 50 g (1⅔ oz) each.

NUTRITIONAL VALUES PER PORTION:
820 Cal • 34 g protein • 48 g fat • 60 g carbohydrate • 9 g dietary fibre • 4 CE

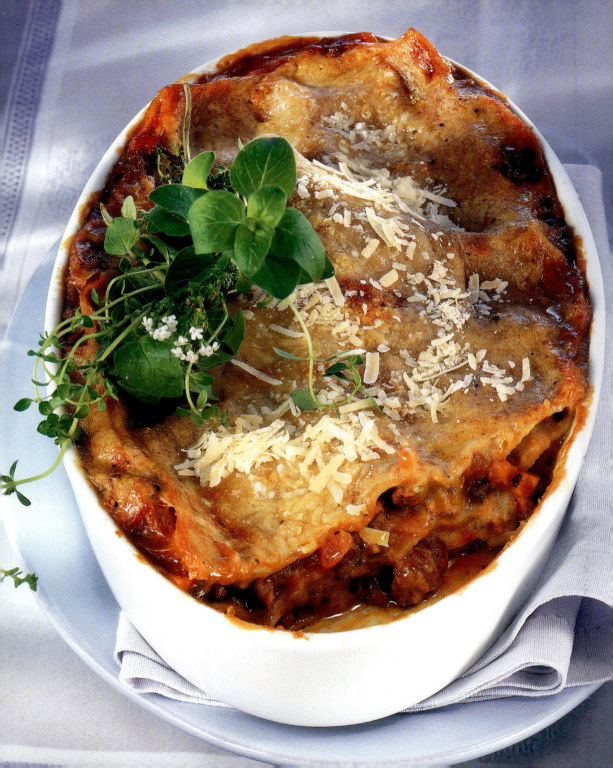

Burgers with roasted vegetables

SERVES 2

FOR THE BURGERS

½ bunch parsley

1 tsp marinated green peppercorns

200 g (6½ oz) lean beef mince

2 tbsp low-fat cream cheese

1 tsp mustard

½ tsp grated lemon zest

1 egg yolk

salt

FOR THE VEGETABLES

1 tbsp olive oil

400 g (13 oz) potatoes

1 small eggplant (aubergine, about 250 g/8 oz)

2 onions

3 small sprigs rosemary

4 sticks celery

100 g (3⅓ oz) small cherry tomatoes

80 ml (2⅔ fl oz/⅓ cup) vegetable stock

pepper

PREPARATION: about 1 hr

1. To make the burgers, wash and pat dry the parsley. Reserving a few leaves for the garnish, chop the rest. Coarsely crush the peppercorns.

2. Combine the minced meat with the cream cheese, mustard, lemon zest, chopped parsley, peppercorns and egg yolk. Season with salt. Shape the minced meat mixture into small burgers or meatballs and chill.

3. Preheat the oven to 200°C (390°F) /180°C (355°F) fan-forced (middle shelf). Brush an ovenproof dish with oil. Peel the potatoes and cut them into eighths. Wash, trim and thickly slice the eggplant. Peel the onions and cut them into eighths. Wash and shake dry the rosemary. Put potatoes, eggplant, onions and rosemary into the dish and cook for about 20 minutes in the oven.

4. Wash and trim the celery, then cut diagonally into 3 cm (1¼ in) lengths, reserving tender green parts. Wash the cherry tomatoes; remove celery tops and set aside. Remove the dish from the oven and add the tomatoes, celery pieces and stock. Stir to combine. Season with salt and pepper. Cook for a further 10–15 minutes.

5. Meanwhile, heat the remaining oil in a non-stick pan and fry the burgers over medium heat for about 4–5 minutes on each side until golden. Chop the remaining celery tops, reserving some for garnishing. Stir into the vegetables. Sprinkle with parsley and celery tops and serve with the burgers.

TIP

Indulge in an entrée or dessert with this main course, depending on your preference and individual carbohydrate requirements. Try for example the Red Jelly with Yoghurt Sauce (see page 112). This dish will supply you with 2 CE per person.

NUTRITIONAL VALUES PER PORTION:

445 Cal • 31 g protein • 24 g fat • 25 g carbohydrate • 9 g dietary fibre • about 1.3 CE

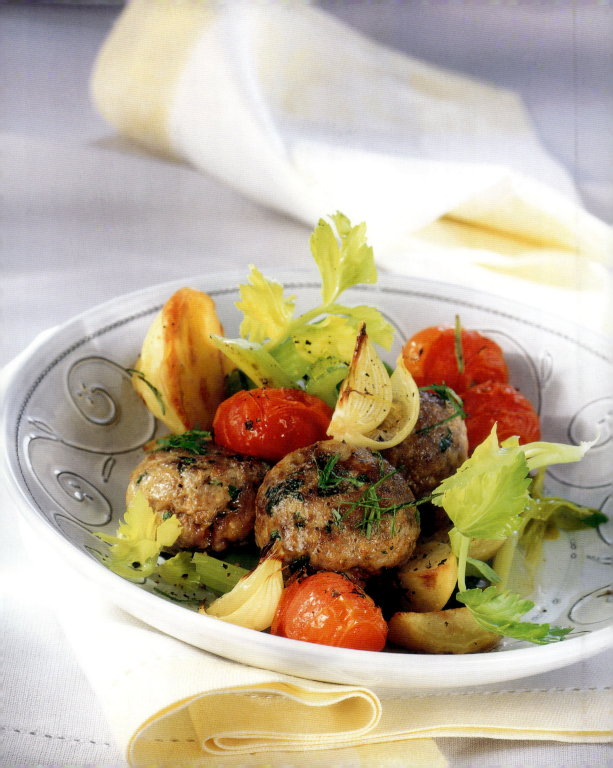

Eggplant Pasta with prosciutto

SERVES 2

1 garlic clove
2 spring onions
2 leaves sage, 2 sprigs thyme
2 sprigs oregano
1 eggplant (aubergine, about 300 g/10 oz)
2 tbsp olive oil
1 tbsp tomato paste
3 tbsp vegetable stock
1 tsp lemon juice
salt, pepper
40 g (1½ oz) prosciutto
150 g (5 oz) wholemeal rigatoni
25 g (¾ oz) grated Parmesan

PREPARATION: about 30 mins

1. Peel and finely dice the garlic. Wash, trim and roughly chop the spring onions. Wash and shake dry the herbs and finely chop the leaves. Wash and trim the eggplant and cut into 1 cm (½ in) pieces.

2. Heat the oil in a non-stick frying pan and fry the eggplant pieces over medium heat for 5 minutes. Add the garlic, spring onions and herbs, and continue frying for 5 minutes. Add the tomato paste and the vegetable stock. Season with lemon juice, salt and pepper. Cover and cook over low heat for about 10 minutes. Cut the prosciutto into strips.

3. Meanwhile, cook the rigatoni in plenty of salted water as per the packet instructions until al dente (firm to the bite). Drain, then combine with the vegetables and half the Parmesan. Arrange the pasta on warmed plates and sprinkle with the prosciutto and the remaining Parmesan.

NUTRITIONAL VALUES PER PORTION:
500 Cal • 23 g protein • 22 g fat • 53 g carbohydrate • 10 g dietary fibre • about 3.3 CE

Venison Medallions with a herb crust

SERVES 2

25 g/¾ oz dried mixed herbs (e.g. parsley, basil, rosemary)
2 tbsp grated Parmesan
1 tbsp wholemeal breadcrumbs
1 tsp horseradish
3 tbsp olive oil
1 large red and 1 large yellow capsicum (pepper)
100 g (3⅓ oz) button mushrooms
2 sprigs thyme
1 small bunch rocket
salt, pepper
4 venison medallions (50 g/1⅔ oz each)
140 g (4½ oz) wholemeal fettucine
5 tbsp vegetable stock

PREPARATION: about 30 mins

1. Whisk together the herbs, the Parmesan, breadcrumbs, horseradish and just under 1 tablespoon oil to make a spreadable paste, adding water, a drop at a time, if necessary.

2. Trim and wash the capsicums, then cut into thin strips. Brush and quarter the mushrooms. Wash and shake dry the thyme and the rocket.

3. Preheat the oven grill. Flatten the medallions a little, season with salt and pepper. Heat 1 tablespoon oil in a frying pan and fry the medallions for 1–2 minutes on each side. Spread with the herb paste and cook under the grill for about 5 minutes. Cook the pasta in plenty of salted water as per the packet instructions until firm to the bite.

4. Meanwhile heat the remaining oil in a pan. Briefly fry the capsicums, mushrooms and thyme. Add the stock; cover and cook briefly so the capsicum stays a little crunchy. Remove from the heat and stir in the rocket. Season with salt and pepper. Drain the pasta. Serve the medallions with the pasta and the vegetables.

> **VARIATION**
> You can replace the venison medallions with pork or beef fillets if you prefer.

NUTRITIONAL VALUES PER PORTION:
615 Cal • 41 g protein • 24 g fat • 58 g carbohydrate • 13 g dietary fibre • 4 CE

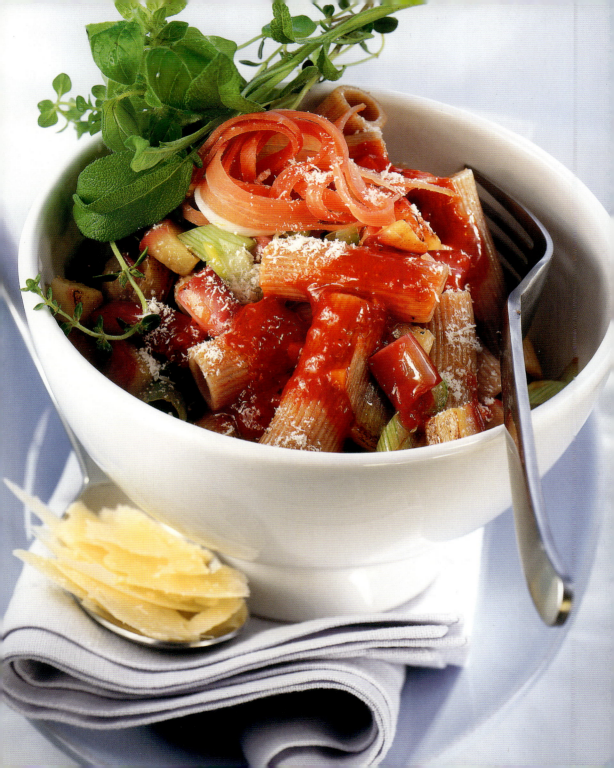

Spicy Lamb Pilaf

SERVES 2

100 g (3⅓ oz) brown rice
300 g (10 oz) lamb (from the leg)
1 onion
250 g (8 oz) tomatoes
1½ tbsp rapeseed oil
salt, pepper
1 pinch ground coriander
½ tsp ground cumin
250 ml (8 fl oz/1 cup) vegetable stock
1 clove
½ bay leaf
1 cinnamon stick (about 4 cm/ 1½ in long)
1 tbsp slivered almonds
½ organic cucumber
2 spring onions
½ tsp lemon juice
150 g yoghurt (3.5% fat)

PREPARATION: about 45 mins
COOKING: about 1 hr

1. Place the rice in a bowl, cover with water and leave to soak for about 15 minutes. Remove any fat and sinew from the lamb; cut the meat into 2 cm (¾ in) dice. Peel and finely chop the onion. Briefly dip the tomatoes in boiling water, peel, then dice.

2. In a saucepan heat 1 tablespoon oil and fry the meat for about 5 minutes to brown all over. Add the onion and fry for a further 2 minutes. Season with salt, pepper, coriander and cumin. Stir in the tomatoes. Turn off the heat and leave the meat to rest for about 10 minutes. Drain the rice.

3. Preheat the oven to 175°C (345°F) /160°C (320°F) fan-forced (middle shelf). Add the rice and stock to the meat. Add the clove, half bay leaf and cinnamon stick, and stir well to combine. Cover and cook in the oven for about 1 hour. Briefly dry-roast the almonds in a non-stick pan without fat.

4. Trim and wash the cucumber, then cut into ½ cm (¼ in) dice. Trim, wash and thinly slice the spring onions. Stir ½ tablespoon oil and the lemon juice into the yoghurt. Stir the cucumber and spring onions into the yoghurt mixture. Season the salad generously with salt and pepper. Sprinkle the pilaf with the almonds. Serve with the cucumber salad.

TIP

It is worth your while to prepare double the amount of pilaf. Freeze the rest or reheat it the next day – it'll be even richer in flavour.

VARIATION

Instead of lamb you can also use lean turkey or chicken for this recipe. If using this meat it will only need about 45 minutes in the oven.

NUTRITIONAL VALUES PER PORTION:
725 Cal • 37 g protein • 43 g fat • 48 g carbohydrate • 3 g dietary fibre • 3 CE

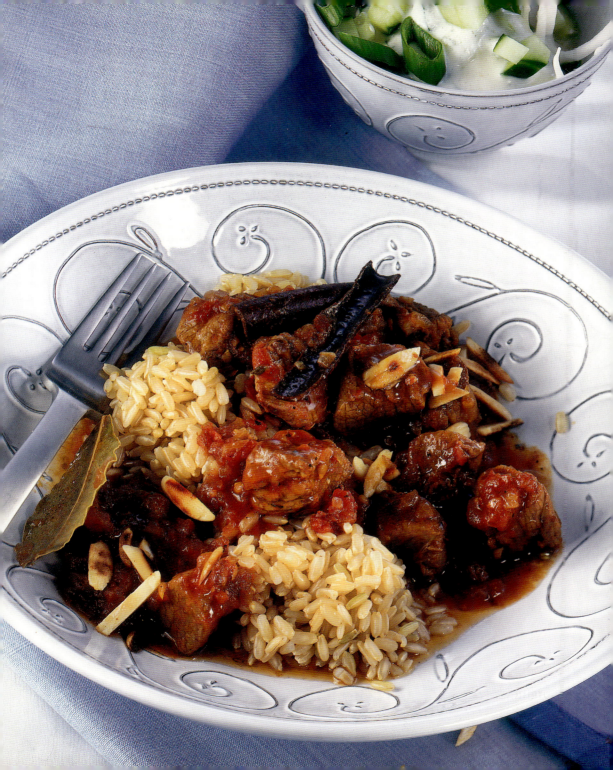

Pancakes with plum compote

SERVES 2 AS A SWEET MAIN COURSE
SERVES 4 AS A DESSERT

FOR THE PANCAKES
50 g (1²/₃ oz) wholemeal spelt flour
125 ml (4 fl oz/½ cup) low-fat milk (1.5% fat)
1 egg
salt
1 tbsp rapeseed oil

FOR THE PLUM COMPOTE
250 g (8 oz) plums
4 tbsp dry red wine (or red grape juice)
1 tbsp sugar
1 pinch ground cinnamon
1 clove
1 small piece of zest from an organic lemon
2 scoops diabetic vanilla ice cream

PREPARATION: about 15 mins
SWELLING: about 30 mins

1. Whisk together the flour, milk, egg and 1 pinch salt to make a pancake batter. Leave covered in the fridge for 30 minutes.

2. Wash, halve and stone the plums. Place the red wine in a saucepan and stir in the sugar. Season with the cinnamon, clove and lemon zest.

3. Heat the red wine mixture. Add the plums, cover and sauté for about 5 minutes. Using a slotted spoon, lift out the plums. Cook the liquid uncovered for about 5 minutes to thicken, until only 3 tablespoons liquid remain.

4. Stir the pancake batter. Heat the oil in a non-stick pan. Bake two pancakes, one at a time.

5. Remove the clove and the lemon zest from the red wine mixture. Fill the pancakes with the plum compote and halve them. Serve drizzled with the red wine sauce and the ice cream.

TIP
These spelt pancakes are delicious as a dessert or as a sweet main course, following a hearty soup or a crunchy salad entrée.

VARIATION
For a change, make a cherry filling for the pancakes. If neither fresh plums nor cherries are available, simply use frozen fruits or preserved fruit from a jar (with artificial sweetener). If you use fruit from a jar, leave the fruit to drain well and reduce the red wine so it thickens straightaway.

NUTRITIONAL VALUES PER PORTION IF MAKING 2 PORTIONS:
365 Cal • 23 g protein • 14 g fat • 44 g carbohydrate • 4 g dietary fibre • about 2.7 CE

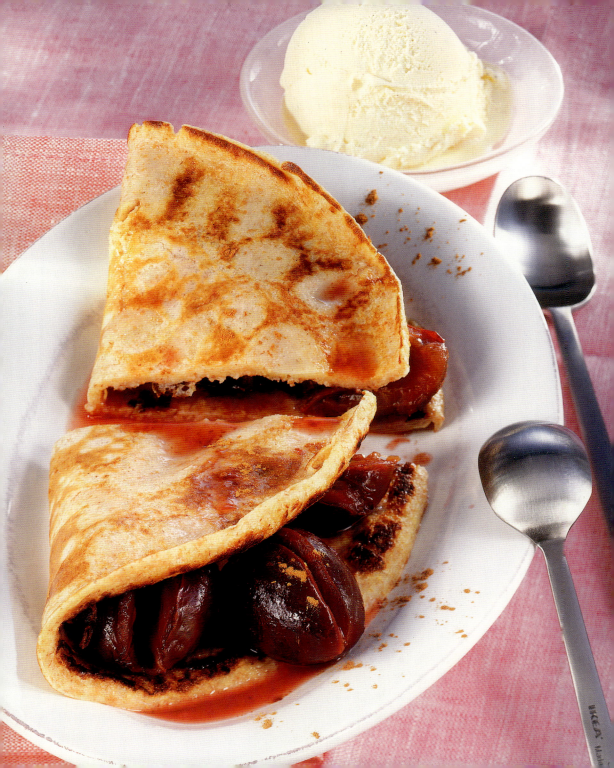

Red Berry Jelly with a yoghurt sauce

SERVES 2
FOR THE JELLY
250 g (8 oz) berries
  (e.g. raspberries, redcurrants
  or strawberries)
¼ tsp agar agar
125 ml (4 fl oz/½ cup) red grape
  juice (unsweetened)
1 tsp lemon juice
1 tbsp sugar
FOR THE SAUCE
150 g (5 oz) yoghurt (3.5% fat)
grated zest of ¼ organic lemon
20 drops liquid sweetener
2 tsp oat bran
PREPARATION: about 15 mins
CHILLING: about 5 hrs

1. Pick over the berries, wash and drain them. Reserve a few nice berries for the garnish. Stir the agar agar into 2 tablespoons grape juice. Bring the remaining juice to the boil together with the lemon juice and the sugar. Stir in the dissolved agar agar and bring the juice back to the boil. Add the berries and bring to the boil again.

2. Turn off the heat and leave the berries in the saucepan for 2 minutes to draw flavour. Divide into individual bowls or cups and chill in the fridge for about 5 hours until the jelly has set.

3. To make the sauce, stir together the yoghurt with the lemon zest, sweetener and oat bran. Divide between serving plates and turn out the jelly. Garnish with the reserved berries and serve.

TIP
If berries are not in season and hard to find, simply use frozen mixed berries for this dish – it'll be just as tasty!

NUTRITIONAL VALUES PER PORTION:
165 Cal • 4 g protein • 3 g fat • 30 g carbohydrate • 4 g dietary fibre • 2 CE

Marinated Peaches with cream cheese

SERVES 2
250 g (8 oz) peaches
1 tbsp lemon juice
1 tbsp sugar
1 pinch ground cardamom
1 tbsp white rum (or orange juice)
4 tbsp freshly pressed orange juice
250 g (8 oz) low-fat cream cheese
1 pinch ground vanilla
½ tsp liquid sweetener
1 tbsp flaked almonds
10 g (½ oz) dark chocolate (with
  at least 70% cocoa)
PREPARATION: about 15 mins

1. Wash, halve and stone the peaches. Cut each half in quarters and drizzle with the lemon juice. Sprinkle over the sugar and cardamom. Stir together the rum and orange juice; marinate the peaches in the mixture.

2. Stir the cream cheese until creamy. Flavour with vanilla and sweetener to taste. Briefly dry-roast the almonds in a non-stick pan without fat; leave to cool. Coarsely grate the chocolate.

3. Divide the peaches between 2 glasses. Set the cream mixture on top. Sprinkle with almonds and chocolate and serve.

TIP
If no fresh peaches are available, use peaches or apricots from the jar (with artificial sweetener) as a substitute. Leave the fruits to drain well and don't add any more sugar.

NUTRITIONAL VALUES PER PORTION:
260 Cal • 19 g protein • 5 g fat • 32 g carbohydrate • 2 g dietary fibre • 2 CE

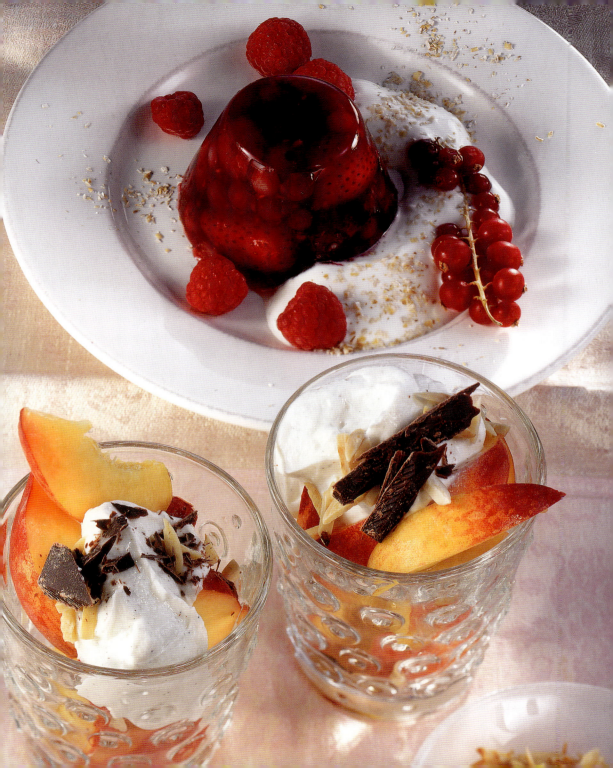

… DESSERTS AND BAKING

Cherry & Pumpernickel Cup

SERVES 2

1 jar sour cherries (morello cherries with artificial sweetener, 185 g/6 oz drained weight)
1 slice pumpernickel (or dark rye bread)
1 tsp grated lemon zest
1 tbsp lemon juice
250 g (8 oz) cream cheese (0.2% fat)
1 tsp fructose
1 pinch ground vanilla

PREPARATION: about 20 mins

1. Leave the cherries to drain well (you could reserve the juice for another dessert).

2. Finely crumble the pumpernickel with your fingertips, then combine with the lemon zest and the lemon juice. Whisk the cream cheese with ½–1 teaspoon fructose and the vanilla.

3. Reserve some of the cherries and a little of the pumpernickel for the garnish. Alternately layer the cream cheese mixture, the remaining cherries and the rest of the pumpernickel into glasses. Garnish with pumpernickel crumbs and cherries. Chill until ready to serve.

BLACK BREAD
Pumpernickel is a German bread made from sourdough and rye. It is cooked for a very long time, which is why it has such a dark, almost black colour. Pumpernickel also has a low glycemic load.

NUTRITIONAL VALUES PER PORTION:
210 Cal • 19 g protein • 1 g fat • 32 g carbohydrate • 3 g dietary fibre • 2 CE

Poached Chocolate Pears

SERVES 2

2 pears (if possible with red skins)
2 tsp lemon juice
50 g (1⅔ oz) dark chocolate (at least 70% cocoa)
100 g (3⅓ oz) red berries (e.g. raspberries, strawberries or redcurrants)

PREPARATION: about 20 mins

1. Wash, then halve the pears, leaving their stem intact. Remove the cores and slice into halves to make a fan shape.

2. Cover the bottom of a frying pan with water. Stir in the lemon juice. Place the pear fans next to each other in the pan and bring the lemon water to the boil. Poach the pear halves for about 3–5 minutes in the liquid.

3. Coarsely chop the chocolate. Place in a bowl set over a saucepan with boiling water to melt, stirring constantly.

4. Lift the pear fans out of the liquid, drain and place 2 fans on each serving plate. Drizzle the liquid chocolate over the top, drawing thin swirls. Pick over the berries, wash and drain them. Garnish the pear fans with the berries and serve.

NUTRITIONAL VALUES PER PORTION:
220 Cal • 2 g protein • 8 g fat • 35 g carbohydrate • 6 g dietary fibre • 2 CE

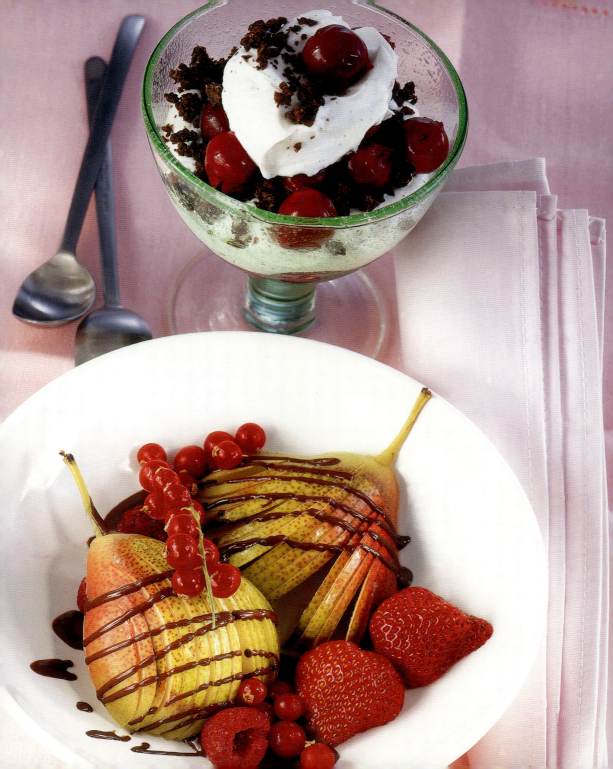

Moroccan Oranges

SERVES 2

2 oranges
1 tsp sesame oil (or rapeseed oil)
1 tsp fructose
1 pinch ground cinnamon
1 pinch ground cloves (or ground allspice)
1 pinch ground vanilla
1 dash white wine (or apple juice)
1 tbsp chopped hazelnuts (or pistachios)

PREPARATION: about 20 mins
MARINATING: 15 MINS

1. Peel the oranges, removing the bitter white pith. Cut the fruit into 1 cm (½ in) slices and halve, catching the juice.

2. In a saucepan, stir together the orange juice and the oil, ½ teaspoon fructose and the spices. Heat through over low heat. Take the spiced liquid off the heat. Add the orange slices, cover and leave to marinate for about 15 minutes, turning once.

3. Lift the orange slices out of the liquid and arrange them on serving plates or bowls. Add the wine to the spiced liquid and briefly bring to the boil. Flavour with the remaining fructose. Leave the liquid to cool a little, then pour over the orange slices. Sprinkle with the chopped hazelnuts and serve.

VARIATION
Instead of the oranges you could also use 1 large pink grapefruit. Peel the fruit, cut the fillets from between the membranes, then halve, catching the juice.

NUTRITIONAL VALUES PER PORTION:
120 Cal • 1 g protein • 6 g fat • 15 g carbohydrate • 2 g dietary fibre • about 1 CE

Strawberry & Tofu Ice Cream

SERVES 2

300 g (10 oz) strawberries (fresh or frozen)
150 g (5 oz) tofu
250 ml (8 fl oz/1 cup) buttermilk
juice of ½ lemon
liquid sweetener
50 g (1⅔ oz) cream

PREPARATION: about 20 mins
FREEZING: 3 HRS

1. If using frozen strawberries, leave to thaw a little. Chop the tofu, then purée with the buttermilk in a food processor at the highest setting or using a hand-held blender. Strain the tofu and buttermilk mixture through a sieve.

2. If using fresh strawberries, wash and hull them. Finely purée the berries, then stir the purée into the tofu and buttermilk mixture. Flavour to taste with lemon juice and sweetener. Whisk the cream until stiff, then fold in.

3. Fill the mixture into portion-sized moulds and freeze for 3 hours. Alternatively, prepare the strawberry ice cream in an ice cream maker. Scoop out the ice cream. Garnish with fresh berries and serve.

VARIATION
You can make raspberry, blackberry or blueberry ice cream in exactly the same way. Garnish with whole fruits to serve.

NUTRITIONAL VALUES PER PORTION:
260 Cal • 12 g protein • 14 g fat • 16 g carbohydrate • 3 g dietary fibre • about 1 CE

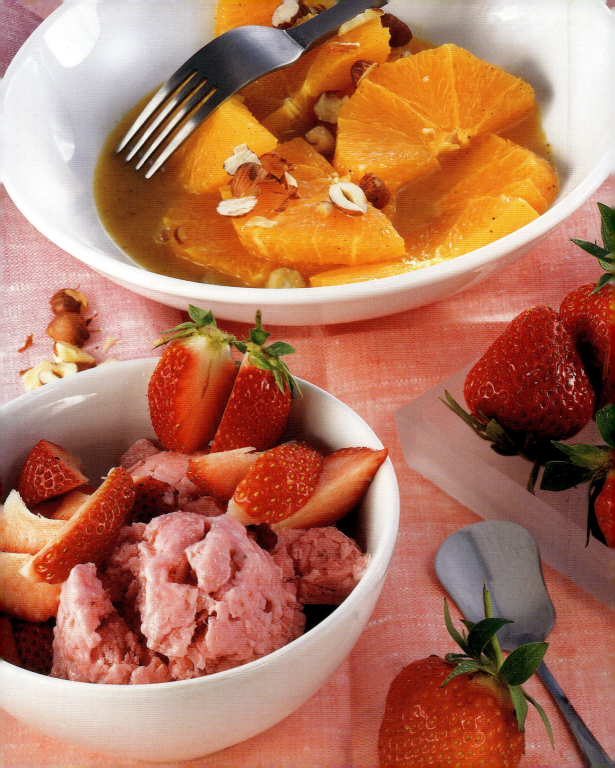

Raspberry Jelly with coconut cream

SERVES 2

300 g (10 oz) frozen raspberries
2 sheets clear gelatine
100 ml (3 fl oz/½ cup) apple juice (unsweetened)
1 tsp lemon juice
liquid sweetener as desired
1 fresh small egg white
3 tbsp cream
2 tsp desiccated coconut (or coconut syrup)
a few lemon balm or mint leaves

PREPARATION: about 20 mins + TIME FOR DEFROSTING
FREEZING: about 2 hrs

1. Leave the raspberries to thaw. Soak the gelatine for 5 minutes in cold water. Purée the thawed raspberries, then push through a fine sieve. Add apple juice to the purée to make up 300 ml (10 fl oz/1¼ cups).

2. Heat 4 tablespoons of the raspberry purée. Dissolve the dripping wet gelatine in the purée, stirring constantly, then stir the mixture into the remaining raspberry purée. Flavour with lemon juice and sweetener to taste. Fill the purée into glasses or dessert bowls and chill for about 2 hours.

3. Just before serving, separately whisk the egg white and the cream until stiff, then gently fold one into the other. Fold in the coconut. Garnish the raspberry jelly with the coconut cream and a few lemon balm leaves and serve.

> **VARIATION**
> You can use this recipe to make a jelly from other frozen berries too. Serve with whipped cream made as per the recipe here.

NUTRITIONAL VALUES PER PORTION:
195 Cal • 6 g protein • 11 g fat • 14 g carbohydrate • 8 g dietary fibre • about 1 CE

Yoghurt & Orange Muffins

MAKES 6 MUFFINS

1 large egg
50 g (1⅔ oz) icing sugar
1 large pinch ground vanilla
grated zest and juice of 1 organic orange
2 tbsp rapeseed oil
50 g (1⅔ oz) low-fat yoghurt (1.5% fat)
125 g (4 oz) wholemeal flour
½ tsp baking powder
2 tbsp ground almonds
1 tbsp yoghurt
2 tsp chopped unsalted pistachios

PREPARATION: about 20 mins
BAKING: about 30 mins

1. Preheat the oven to 180°C (355°F) /160°C (320°F) fan-forced (middle shelf). Place 2 paper cases inside each other for each muffin. Whisk the egg with the icing sugar, vanilla, orange zest, 4 tablespoons orange juice, oil and yoghurt until combined. Combine the flour with the baking powder and the almonds, then fold into the egg mixture.

2. Fill the dough into the paper cases and bake in the oven for about 25 minutes. Leave the muffins to cool. Just before serving, stir the yoghurt until smooth. Place a dollop on each muffin and sprinkle the pistachios on top.

> **VARIATION**
> You can replace the orange with 1 small untreated lemon or 1 lime, if you like. Finely grate the zest and squeeze out the juice.

NUTRITIONAL VALUES PER PORTION:
175 Cal • 5 g protein • 7 g fat • 24 g carbohydrate • 1 g dietary fibre • about 1.3 CE

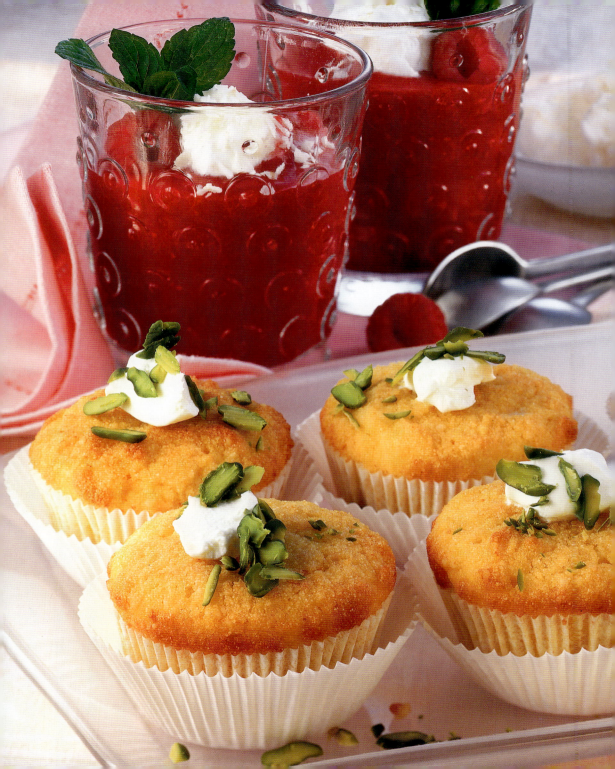

Cream Cheese Croissants with poppy seeds

MAKES 8 CROISSANTS
FOR THE DOUGH
125 g (4 oz) low-fat cream cheese
2 tbsp low-fat milk (1.5% fat)
1 egg
2 tbsp sugar
salt
4 tbsp corn oil
250 g (8 oz) wholemeal flour
¾ tsp baking powder
FOR THE FILLING
125 g (4 oz) low-fat cream cheese
2 tbsp poppy seeds
grated zest of ¼ organic lemon
1 large pinch ground vanilla
½ tsp liquid sweetener
flour, for dusting
PLUS
1 tbsp condensed milk
20 g (⅔ oz) chopped hazelnuts
1 tbsp sugar
PREPARATION: about 20 mins
RESTING: 30 mins
BAKING: 25 mins

1. To make the dough, stir the cream cheese, milk, egg, sugar, 1 pinch salt and the oil together until smooth. Combine the flour with the baking powder and sift over the cream cheese mixture. Knead, initially using the dough hook of the hand-held blender, then with your hands. If the dough is too crumbly, knead in a few drops of water. Wrap in cling film and leave to rest at room temperature for about 30 minutes.

2. To make the filling, drain the cream cheese. Lightly crush the poppy seeds in a mortar and pestle. Stir the lemon zest, the vanilla and the sweetener into the cream cheese.

3. Preheat the oven to 200°C (390°F) /180°C (355°F) fan-forced (middle shelf). Line a baking tray with baking paper. On a floured work surface, roll out the dough to a circle of 35 cm (14 in) diameter. Spread the poppy seeds on top and cut the circle into eighths.

4. Put roughly 1 teaspoon cream cheese filling on top of each eighth and spread evenly. Now roll up from the wide side towards the tip to form croissants. Combine hazelnuts and sugar. Brush the croissants with condensed milk, sprinkle with the nut mixture and place on the baking tray. Bake in the oven for about 25 minutes.

TIP

These croissants are at their tastiest when eaten fresh from the oven. Whatever is left over can be frozen. To serve, just bake the frozen croissants for 10 minutes, until they are crisp again.

NUTRITIONAL VALUES PER PORTION:
230 Cal • 10 g protein • 9 g fat • 27 g carbohydrate • 5 g dietary fibre • about 1.7 CE

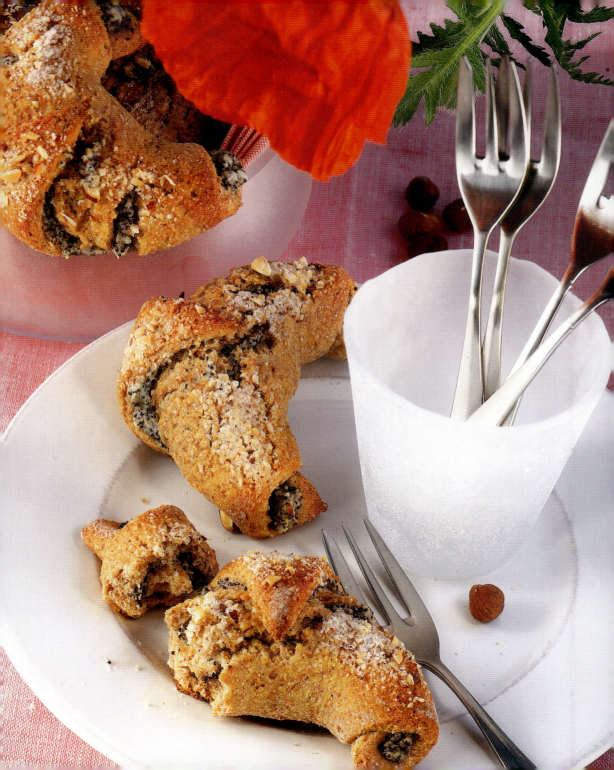

Cinnamon Apple Crumble

SERVES 2
400 g (13 oz) cooking apples
1 tbsp lemon juice
50 ml (2 fl oz/¼ cup) apple juice (unsweetened)
30 g (1 oz) wholemeal flour
25 g (¾ oz) soft margarine
1 tbsp chopped walnuts
1 tbsp coarse wholemeal oats
¼ tsp ground cinnamon
1 pinch ground cloves
1 heaped tbsp sugar
PREPARATION: about 15 mins
BAKING: about 15 mins

1. Wash, quarter and core the apples, then drizzle with the lemon juice. Bring the apple juice to the boil. Add the apples, cover and simmer for about 5 minutes.

2. Preheat the oven to 200°C (390°F) /180°C (355°F) fan-forced (middle shelf). Knead together the flour and the margarine. Add the walnuts, oats, cinnamon, cloves and half the sugar, and knead with your fingertips to form a crumble.

3. Place the apples and juice in an ovenproof dish. Spread the crumble on top and sprinkle with the remaining sugar. Bake in the oven for about 15 minutes until golden. Serve hot.

TIP
Instead of ordinary household sugar, use an unrefined cane sugar – it has a very pleasant flavour similar to caramel.

NUTRITIONAL VALUES PER PORTION:
340 Cal • 3 g protein • 14 g fat • 50 g carbohydrate • 7 g dietary fibre • about 3.3 CE

Cheesecake with apricots

MAKES 6 PIECES
400 g (13 oz) low-fat cream cheese
2 eggs
50 g (1²⁄₃ oz) soft margarine
grated zest of ½ organic lemon
1 large pinch ground vanilla
50 g (1²⁄₃ oz) wholemeal semolina
½ tsp baking powder
1 tsp liquid sweetener
butter and breadcrumbs, for greasing
250 g (8 oz) apricots
1 tbsp lemon juice
salt
PREPARATION: about 20 mins
BAKING: about 45 mins

1. Drain the cream cheese. Separate the eggs. Whisk the margarine, lemon zest, vanilla and egg yolks. Combine the semolina and the baking powder. Stir into the egg yolk mixture along with the cream cheese and the sweetener.

2. Preheat the oven to 200°C (390°F) /180°C (355°F) fan-forced (middle shelf). Grease a loose-bottomed tin (18 cm/7 in diameter) and sprinkle with breadcrumbs. Wash, halve and stone the apricots. Drizzle with the lemon juice.

3. Beat the egg whites with a pinch salt until stiff, then fold into the cream cheese mixture. Fill into the tin, cover with the apricots. Bake for 45 minutes. Leave in the tin to cool.

TIP
If fresh apricots are not in season, you can use preserved apricots from a jar instead (with artificial sweetener). Make sure you drain the fruit well before using.

NUTRITIONAL VALUES PER PORTION:
220 Cal • 13 g protein • 12 g fat • 14 g carbohydrate • 1 g dietary fibre • about 1 CE

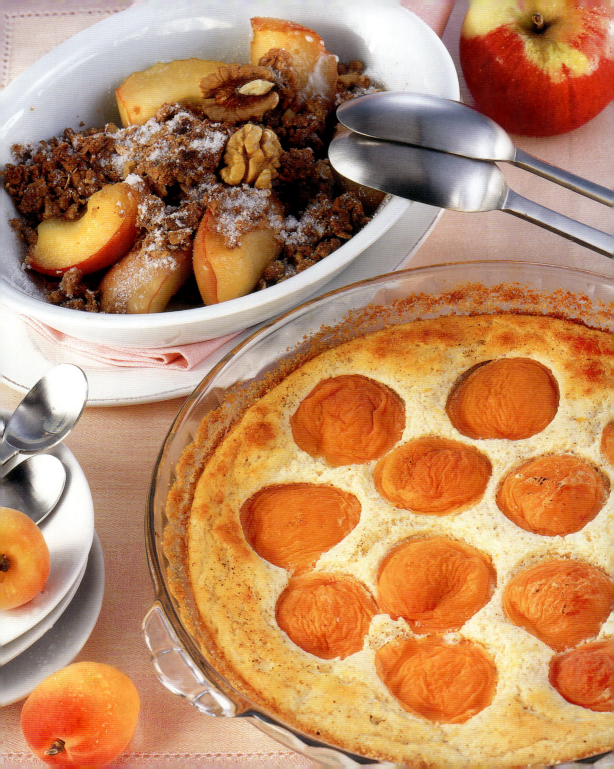

THE FOOD PYRAMID

THE AUSTRALIAN DIABETES ASSOCIATION recommend maintaining a healthy balance of nutrients. The healthy foods pyramid on the right clearly indicates the basis for these recommendations. The wider the base of the individual food groups, the greater the quantities of these foods that should be incorporated into your daily menu plan.

CARBOHYDRATE

CHOOSE WHOLEMEAL
Choose wholemeal products if you can, and as little processed cereal products as possible, for carbohydrates play a central role in your metabolism. An adult will "use up" approximately 180 g (5¾ oz) carbohydrate within 24 hours in order to supply the brain, the nerves, the red blood cells and the kidneys. By eating sufficient carbohydrate, of the "right" sort, you can avoid low blood sugar values, reduction in performance, loss of concentration and food cravings. Good carbohydrate-rich foods also contain many vitamins, minerals and dietary fibre. Cereals and cereal products as well as potatoes are all good sources of carbohydrates.

EAT FRESH FRUIT AND VEGETABLES OFTEN
Fresh sweet fruit contains natural sugar. Enjoy up to three serves a day (up to 200 g/6½ oz, depending on the variety). You can eat fresh vegetables and salads to your heart's content. Vegetables in serves up to 200 g (6½ oz) are not counted. Vegetables and salads are great sources of essential nutrients, yet they are very low in calories.

LITTLE EXTRAS
Sugar, sugary drinks, sweets, pastries and products made from plain flour supply carbohydrates in a concentrated form – without the additional vital nutrients and often with a high glycemic index. Sweets and plain flour products are therefore not forbidden; however, you should indulge in such foods only occasionally and in small quantities. When you do, make sure you enjoy them. The same applies to alcoholic drinks.

PROTEIN AND FAT

This is the way to give your body a sufficient and balanced supply of quality proteins, essential fatty acids and energy: in preference, choose low-fat milk, milk products and cheese varieties. You can eat meat dishes two to three times a week, but make sure you choose dark (muscle) meat and poultry pieces without skin in preference to fatty cuts. Fish should feature at least six times on your monthly menu plan. Be certain to include oily fish such as herring, salmon, mackerel and tuna – these supply unsaturated and omega-3 fatty acids, which are often lacking in our diet but are of vital importance to our health. Quality oils, especially oils made from rapeseed, olives and walnuts, should – in small quantities – feature daily on your menu plan.

USE SPARINGLY
Hydrogenated margarine and plant-based fats, butter, fatty meats and cold cuts, ready-made foods, sweets, baked goods and "extra creamy" products supply the body only with "lazy" instead of healthy fatty acids – thereby further increasing the need for unsaturated fats. It is best if you consume these foods in small quantities only. Nuts, however, supply high-quality fatty acids, proteins and many minerals. They are packed with lots of energy-giving nutrients, however, you are still advised to indulge in only a handful of nuts a week.

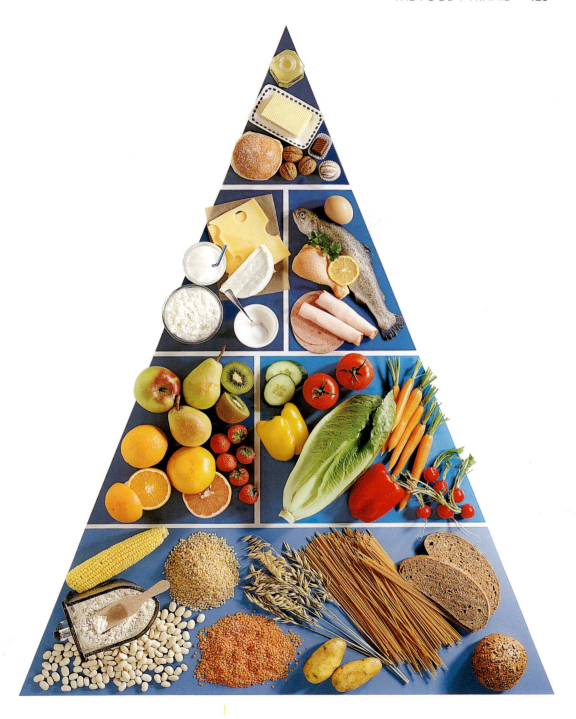

Delicious meals for type 2 diattics – the first week at a glance

What your first weekly diet plan might look like (12 CE per day)	Breakfast 1	Breakfast 2
Day 1	zucchini scrambled eggs (p. 32) 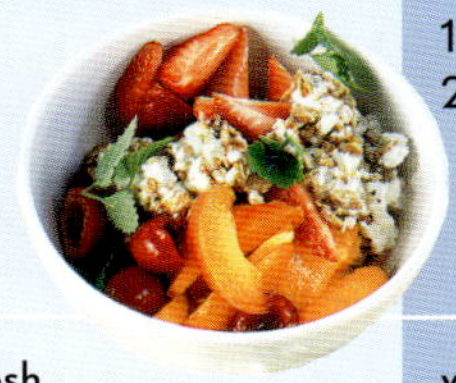	1 small apple and 250 g (8 oz) plain yoghurt
Day 2	muesli with fresh fruit (p. 24)	vegetable drink (p. 36) and 4 pumpernickel rounds (10 g/½ oz each)
Day 3	bread roll with basil tofu (p. 28)	150 g (5 oz) grapes and 200 ml (7 fl oz/¾ cup) buttermilk
Day 4	apple & cream cheese sandwich (p. 29) 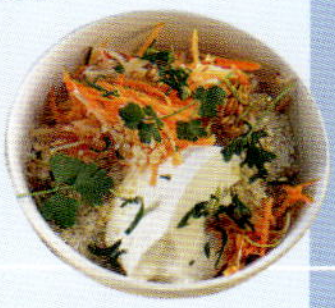	200 ml (7 fl oz/¾ cup) vegetable juice and 3 pumpernickel rounds (10 g/½ oz each)
Day 5	hearty millet muesli (p. 27)	1 medium pear and 200 ml (7 fl oz/¾ cup) buttermilk
Day 6	cheese & apricot open sandwich (p. 29)	Indian Lassi (p. 36) and 2 nectarines
Day 7	fresh grain muesli (p. 26) 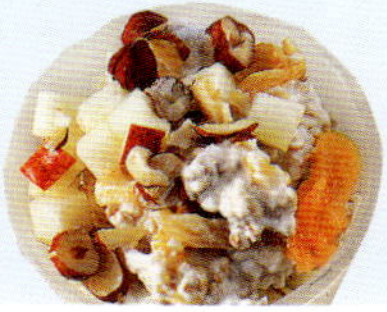	vanilla & ginger tea (p. 37) and 1 orange

WEEKLY DIET PLAN

Lunch	Afternoon	Dinner	Supper
millet with ratatouille (p. 64)	vanilla & ginger tea (p. 37)	chicory & grape salad (p. 40)	shake: 250 g (8 oz) plain yoghurt and 200 g (6½ oz) berries
cod with leek and tomatoes (p. 80)	1 apple	Cheese and salad rolls (p. 33)	shake: 200 ml (7 fl oz/¾ cup) buttermilk and 1 small banana
spinach-filled cannelloni (p. 68)	cheese & vegetable snack (p. 32) and wholemeal bread	chickpea salad with herb dressing (p. 42)	100 g (3⅓ oz) cottage cheese and 1 nectarine
vegetable rice with hard-boiled eggs (p. 62)	Moroccan oranges (p. 116)	fennel & tomatoes with Parmesan (p. 56)	mix: 125 g (4 oz) low-fat cream cheese + 200 g (6½ oz) raspberries
ocean perch ragout (p. 86)	200 ml (7 fl oz/¾ cup) vegetable juice, 3 pumpernickel rounds (10 g/½ oz each)	savoury baked apples (p. 60)	100 g (3⅓ oz) cottage cheese and 120 g (4 oz) orange
wok vegetables with glass noodles (p. 72) and 1 yoghurt & orange muffin (p. 118)	1 medium pear	barley & vegetable soup (p. 46)	mix: 125 g (4 oz) low-fat cream cheese + 1 tbsp yoghurt + 200 g (6½ oz) raspberries
chicken breast with pineapple (p. 98)	1 yoghurt & orange muffin (p. 118)	broccoli with walnuts (p. 52)	mix: 125 g (4 oz) plain yoghurt + 1 small puréed banana

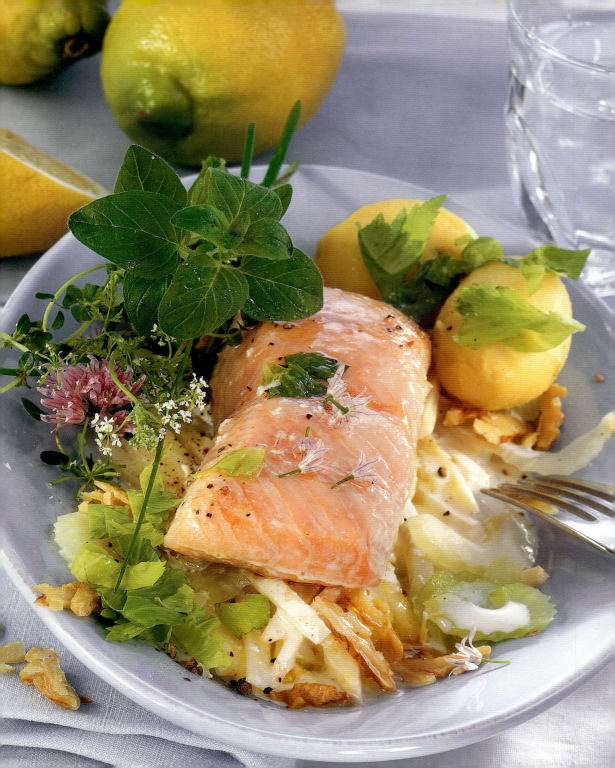

RECIPES INDEX – BY CHAPTER

BREAKFAST, SNACKS AND DRINKS
apple & coconut porridge 27
apple & cream cheese open sandwich 29
bread roll with basil tofu 28
capsicum boats with tzatziki 33
cheese & apricot open sandwich 29
cheese & salad rolls 33
cheese & vegetable snack 32
citrus fruit muesli 26
corned beef open sandwich 28
eggplant spread with capsicum 31
fresh grain muesli 26
ham rolls with radishes 34
hearty millet muesli 27
herring salad on wholegrain bread 34
hummus with sesame seeds 30
Indian lassi 36
muesli with fresh fruit 24
olive & roasted vegetable paste 31
peach frappé with cream 37
vanilla & ginger tea 37
vegetable drink 36
zucchini scrambled eggs 32

SNACKS AND STARTERS
Asian vegetable soup 50
barley & vegetable soup 46
bean salad with tuna 38
broccoli with nuts 52
cauliflower with a curried yoghurt sauce 54
cheesy zucchini parcels 60
chickpea salad with herb dressing 42
chicory & grape salad with cheese dressing 40
couscous salad 42
eggplant bake 58
fennel & tomatoes with Parmesan 56

French onion soup 48
Jerusalem artichoke soup 48
kohlrabi & potato bake 58
Mediterranean vegetables 54
Moroccan carrot salad 44
orange salad with onions 45
quick tomato soup 50
red lentil soup with parsley oil 46
savoury baked apples 60
vegetable salad with yoghurt 45
warm radicchio salad 52
warm savoy cabbage salad 40

MAIN COURSES – VEGETARIAN
cabbage rolls with bulgur filling 66
fried vegetables with parsley sauce 72
lentil rice with vegetables 76
millet with ratatouille 64
pizza with artichokes 70
spaghetti with pumpkin seed & herb pesto 68
spinach dumplings with tomato sauce 64
spinach-filled cannelloni 68
spinach in a sesame sauce 56
turnip quiche 74
vegetable rice with hard-boiled eggs 62
wok vegetables with glass noodles 72

MAIN COURSES – WITH FISH
barramundi & vegetables 92
barramundi in an olive and caper sauce 84
capsicum barley with prawns 88
cod with leek and tomatoes 80
fish fillets in a sesame crust 82
fish kebabs with lemon sauce 84
fish osso buco 92
fish with panfried mushrooms 80
ling fillet in a cheese & vegetable crust 88

mackerel baked in foil 78
ocean perch ragout 86
salmon on Waldorf salad 90

MAIN COURSES – WITH POULTRY
chicken breast with pineapple 98
Creole chicken casserole 94
curried turkey strips 96
duck breast with broccoli and nuts 98
filled turkey rolls 96
lemon chicken 100
oven-baked turkey drumstick 100

MAIN COURSES – WITH MEAT
burgers with roasted vegetables 104
eggplant pasta with prosciutto 106
lasagne with meat & vegetables 102
spicy lamb pilaf 108
venison medallions with a herb crust 106

DESSERTS AND BAKING
cheesecake with apricots 122
cherry & pumpernickel cup 114
cinnamon apple crumble 122
cream cheese croissants with poppy seeds 120
marinated peaches with cream cheese 112
Moroccan oranges 116
pancakes with plum compote 110
poached chocolate pears 114
raspberry jelly with coconut cream 118
red berry jelly with a yoghurt sauce 112
strawberry & tofu ice cream 116
yoghurt & orange muffins 118

INDEX

Apples
    apple & coconut porridge 27
    apple & cream cheese open
        sandwich 29
    cinnamon apple crumble 122
    hearty millet muesli 27
    salmon on Waldorf salad 90
    savoury baked apples 60
apple & coconut porridge 27
apple & cream cheese open sandwich 29
Asian vegetable soup 50

Baked goods
    cheesecake with apricots 122
    cinnamon apple crumble 122
    cream cheese croissants with
        poppy seeds 120
    yoghurt & orange muffins 118
barley & vegetable soup 46
barramundi & vegetables 92
barramundi in an olive and caper sauce 84
bean salad with tuna 38
Berry fruit
    strawberry & tofu ice cream 116
    raspberry jelly w. coconut cream 118
    muesli with fresh fruit 24
    red berry jelly with a yoghurt sauce 112
Bread and bread rolls
    apple & cream cheese open sandwich 29
    bread roll with basil tofu 28
    cheese & apricot open sandwich 29
    cheese & salad rolls 33
    corned beef open sandwich 28
    ham rolls with radishes 34
    herring salad on wholegrain bread 34
bread roll with basil tofu 28
Broccoli
    broccoli with nuts 52
    duck breast w. broccoli & nuts 98
    fish kebabs with lemon sauce 84
    fried vegetables w. parsley sauce 72
broccoli with nuts 52
burgers with roasted vegetables 104

cabbage rolls with bulgur filling 66
Capsicum
    barramundi & vegetables 92
    capsicum barley with prawns 88

    capsicum boats with tzatziki 33
    cheese & salad rolls 33
    chicken breast with pineapple 98
    Creole chicken casserole 94
    eggplant spread with capsicum 31
    Mediterranean vegetables 54
    millet with ratatouille 64
    ocean perch ragout 86
    warm savoy cabbage salad 40
    wok vegetables with glass noodles 72
capsicum barley with prawns 88
capsicum boats with tzatziki 33
Carrots
    couscous salad 42
    fried vegetables with parsley sauce 72
    hearty millet muesli 27
    Jerusalem artichoke soup 48
    mackerel baked in foil 78
    Moroccan carrot salad 44
    oven-baked turkey drumstick 100
    vegetable rice with hard-boiled eggs 62
Cauliflower
    cauliflower with a curried yoghurt sauce 54
    lentil rice with vegetables 76
    cauliflower with a curried yoghurt sauce 54
Cheese
    cheese & vegetable snack 32
    cheesy zucchini parcels 60
    eggplant bake 58
    eggplant pasta w. prosciutto 106
    fennel & tomatoes with Parmesan 56
    French onion soup 48
    lasagne with meat & vegetables 102
    ling fillet in a cheese & vegetable crust 88
    pizza with artichokes 70
    turnip quiche 74
    warm radicchio salad 52
cheese & apricot open sandwich 29
cheese & salad rolls 33
cheese & vegetable snack 32
cheesecake with apricots 122
cheesy zucchini parcels 60
cherry & pumpernickel cup 114
chicken breast with pineapple 98
chickpea salad w. herb dressing 42
chicory & grape salad with cheese

    dressing 40
cinnamon apple crumble 122
citrus fruit muesli 26
cod with leek and tomatoes 80
corned beef open sandwich 28
couscous salad 42
cream cheese croissants with
    poppy seeds 120
Creole chicken casserole 94
curried turkey strips 96

Desserts
    marinated peaches with cream cheese 112
    Moroccan oranges 116
    pancakes with plum compote 110
    poached chocolate pears 114
    raspberry jelly with coconut cream 118
    red berry jelly with a yoghurt sauce 112
    strawberry & tofu ice cream 116
Drinks
    Indian lassi 36
    peach frappé with cream 37
    vanilla & ginger tea 37
    vegetable drink 36
duck breast with broccoli & nuts 98

Eggplant
    burgers with roasted vegetables 104
    eggplant spread with capsicum 31
    eggplant pasta with prosciutto 106
    eggplant bake 58
    millet with ratatouille 64
eggplant bake 58
eggplant pasta with prosciutto 106
eggplant spread with capsicum 31

Fennel
    cheese & salad rolls 33
    fennel & tomatoes with Parmesan 56
    mackerel baked in foil 78
    Mediterranean vegetables 54
    fennel & tomatoes with Parmesan 56
filled turkey rolls 96
fish fillets in a sesame crust 82
fish kebabs with lemon sauce 84
fish osso buco 92
fish with panfried mushrooms 80
French onion soup 48

INDEX

fresh grain muesli 26
fried vegetables with parsley sauce 72

ham rolls with radishes 34
hearty millet muesli 27
herring salad on wholegrain bread 34
hummus with sesame seeds 30

Indian lassi 36

Jerusalem artichoke soup 48

kohlrabi & potato bake 58

lasagne with meat & vegetables 102
lemon chicken 100
lentil rice with vegetables 76
ling fillet in a cheese & vegetable crust 88

mackerel baked in foil 78
marinated peaches with cream cheese 112
Mediterranean vegetables 54
millet with ratatouille 64
Moroccan carrot salad 44
Moroccan oranges 116
Muesli
   citrus fruit muesli 26
   fresh grain muesli 26
   hearty millet muesli 27
   muesli with fresh fruit 24
muesli with fresh fruit 24
Mushrooms
   fish with panfried mushrooms 80
   fried vegetables with parsley sauce 72
   mackerel baked in foil 78
   venison medallions with a herb crust 106

ocean perch ragout 86
olive & roasted vegetable paste 31
Oranges
   Moroccan oranges 116
   ocean perch ragout 86
   orange salad with onions 45
   yoghurt & orange muffins 118
orange salad with onions 45
oven-baked turkey drumstick 100

pancakes with plum compote 110

Pasta
   barramundi in an olive and caper sauce 84
   eggplant pasta w. prosciutto 106
   lasagne with meat and vegetables 102
   spaghetti with pumpkin seed & herb pesto 68
   spinach-filled cannelloni 68
peach frappé with cream 37
pizza with artichokes 70
poached chocolate pears 114
Potatoes
   burgers with roasted vegetables 104
   Creole chicken casserole 94
   fried vegetables with parsley sauce 72
   kohlrabi & potato bake 58
   kohlrabi quiche 74
   oven-baked turkey drumstick 100
   salmon on Waldorf salad 90

quick tomato soup 50

raspberry jelly w. coconut cream 118
red berry jelly w. yoghurt sauce 112
red lentil soup with parsley oil 46
Rice
   lentil rice with vegetables 76
   spicy lamb pilaf 108
   vegetable rice with hard-boiled eggs 62

Salads
   bean salad with tuna 38
   chickpea salad with herb dressing 42
   chicory & grape salad with cheese dressing 40
   couscous salad 42
   Moroccan carrot salad 44
   orange salad with onions 45
   vegetable salad with yoghurt 45
   warm radicchio salad 52
   warm savoy cabbage salad 40
   salmon on Waldorf salad 90
savoury baked apples 60
Soups
   Asian vegetable soup 50
   barley & vegetable soup 46
   French onion soup 48
   Jerusalem artichoke soup 48
   quick tomato soup 50
   red lentil soup with parsley oil 46
spaghetti with pumpkin seed & herb pesto 68
spicy lamb pilaf 108
Spinach

spinach dumplings with tomato sauce 64
spinach-filled cannelloni 68
spinach in a sesame sauce 56
spinach dumplings with tomato sauce 64
spinach-filled cannelloni 68
spinach in a sesame sauce 56
Spreads
   eggplant spread with capsicum 31
   hummus with sesame seeds 30
   olive & roasted vegetable paste 31
strawberry & tofu ice cream 116

Tomatoes
   bread roll with basil tofu 28
   burgers w. roasted vegetables 104
   cheese & vegetable snack 32
   chickpea salad with herb dressing 42
   cod with leek and tomatoes 80
   couscous salad 42
   fennel & tomatoes with Parmesan 56
   filled turkey rolls 96
   quick tomato soup 50
   pizza with artichokes 70
   spicy lamb pilaf 108
   spinach dumplings with tomato sauce 64
   spinach-filled cannelloni 68
turnip quiche 74

vanilla & ginger tea 37
vegetable drink 36
vegetable rice w. hard-boiled eggs 62
vegetable salad with yoghurt 45
venison medallions with a herb crust 106

warm radicchio salad 52
warm savoy cabbage salad 40
wok vegetables w. glass noodles 72

yoghurt & orange muffins 118

Zucchini
   barramundi & vegetables 92
   cheesy zucchini parcels 60
   Creole chicken casserole 94
   ling fillet in a cheese & vegetable crust 88
   millet with ratatouille 64
   vegetable salad with yoghurt 45
   zucchini scrambled eggs 32

This edition published in 2015 by New Holland Publishers Pty Ltd
London • Sydney • Auckland

Unit 9, The Chandlery, 50 Westminster Bridge Road, London SE1 7QY, United Kingdom
1/66 Gibbes Street, Chatswood, NSW 2067, Australia
218 Lake Road, Northcote, Auckland 0627, New Zealand

www.newhollandpublishers.com

Copyright © 2015 New Holland Publishers Pty Ltd
Copyright © 2015 in text: Marlisa Szwillus and Doris Fritzsche
Copyright © 2015 in images: p. 4/5, p. 22/23: Jörn Rynio, Hamburg
all others: Studio L'EVEQUE, Munich, Germany

Published originally under the title Healthy Recipes for Type 2 Diabetics by Marlisa Szwillus and Doris Fritzsche (ISBN 3-7742-6650) © 2004 by GRÄFE UND UNZER VERLAG GmbH, München
English translation copyright: © 2012 by Silva Editions Ltd., France.

All rights reserved. No part of this publication may be reproduced, stored in a retrieval system or transmitted, in any form or by any means, electronic, mechanical, photocopying, recording or otherwise, without the prior written permission of the publishers and copyright holders.

A record of this book is held at the British Library and the National Library of Australia.
ISBN 9781742576312

DISCLAIMER: The nutritional information for each recipe is an estimate only and may vary depending on the brand of ingredients used and due to natural biological variations in the composition of natural foods such as meat, fish, fruit and vegetables. All information provided in this book is intended to be a guide only, it does not replace medical advice. Any concerns readers have about their diet should be discussed with their doctor. Whilst all reasonable efforts have been made to ensure the accuracy of the information, the Publisher accepts no responsibility for the accuracy of that information or for any error or omission and shall not be responsible for any decisions made based on such information.

Managing Director: Fiona Schultz
Publisher: Alan Whiticker
Project Editor: Angela Sutherland
Designer: Thomas Casey
Production Director: Olga Dementiev
Printer: Toppan Leefung Printing Ltd

10 9 8 7 6 5 4 3 2 1

Keep up with New Holland Publishers on Facebook
www.facebook.com/NewHollandPublishers